WOMEN

OF THE

PANDEMIC

ALSO BY LAUREN McKEON

No More Nice Girls

F-Bomb

LAUREN McKEON

WOMEN
OF THE
PANDEMIC

Stories from the
Front Lines of COVID-19

McClelland & Stewart

First edition published 2021

McClelland & Stewart and colophon are registered trademarks of
Penguin Random House Canada Limited.

Library and Archives Canada Cataloguing in Publication data
is available upon request.

ISBN: 978-0-7710-5039-8
ebook ISBN: 978-0-7710-5048-0

Book design by Andrew Roberts
Cover images: (faces) adamkaz / Getty Images; (woman) Olga Maloushkina /
Shutterstock Images; (lettering) Julia August / Shutterstock Images
Typeset in Warnock by M&S, Toronto
Printed and bound in Canada

McClelland & Stewart,
a division of Penguin Random House Canada Limited,
a Penguin Random House Company
www.penguinrandomhouse.ca

1 2 3 4 5   25 24 23 22 21

Penguin
Random House
McCLELLAND & STEWART

To all the women on the front line—thank you.

Contents

WOMEN
OF THE
PANDEMIC

Introduction

In early December 2019, the Huanan Seafood Wholesale Market in Wuhan was bustling. Customers wove their way through the narrowly spaced stalls, shrewdly eyeing coils of octopus, slabs of fat-laced meat, pyramids of fresh greens. It's possible they bought a freshly slaughtered animal: tuna, deer, hedgehog, something else. In certain areas, their shoes likely sloshed through the water vendors use to constantly hose down produce, fish, and other perishable goods, giving the nickname "wet market" to such places in China and other countries across Asia. Maybe their fingertips brushed a stranger's hand as they browsed, or when they paid, or through any other simple accident. Or perhaps none of that happened before they went home to families, groceries in hand, ready to cook dinner, ready to relax. Months later, science was still unable to definitively explain what separated the first unlucky group—twenty-seven market vendors, employees, and customers—from everyone else in Wuhan, including at least a dozen others who suddenly arrived in the city's hospitals that month with mysterious pneumonia-like symptoms.

It didn't take long for doctors and researchers in China to realize the puzzling virus was new, highly contagious, and deadly. The Wuhan Municipal Health Commission announced the potential SARS-like illness to media in late December. In less than a week, the number of cases climbed from forty-one to fifty-nine. Then, on January 11, a sixty-one-year-old man who was a regular customer at the market died. He had been admitted to the hospital after a seven-day fever, persistent cough, and difficulty breathing. Five days after he became sick, his fifty-three-year-old wife, who'd never been to the market, was also admitted. Still, at the time, few fully grasped the wildfire nature of the yet-unnamed novel coronavirus. By January 19, both the Chinese government and the World Health Organization (WHO) had estimated the virus had only "limited" potential for human-to-human transmission. Four days later, China abruptly closed Wuhan's borders, shutting off transportation both to/from and within the city. Seventeen people had died, and at least another 570 were sick.

A week after that, the WHO declared a global health emergency. "If [China] fails to control it, then we should also be grateful to them, because they have demonstrated that it cannot be controlled," Dr. Allison McGeer, an infectious disease specialist at Mount Sinai Hospital in Toronto, told media that same day. "If these public health measures are not enough, then none of the rest of us will be able to do it either." People were worried the virus could be another SARS (Severe Acute Respiratory Syndrome), which has, to date, killed 800 people worldwide, or MERS (Middle East Respiratory Syndrome), which has not been eradicated and which had, by the end of 2019, killed over 850 people. McGeer, who had been on the front lines of the SARS fight, and who had herself contracted the virus, repeatedly assured media that, for now, for Canadians, the virus wasn't anything to worry about. "There are things that should frighten you about this coronavirus," she added, "but getting it in Toronto today is not one of them." Still, she cautioned, the modern world had never before watched the emergence of a new virus. Like other medical experts, she urged calm. In North America, the dominant refrain took shape: This virus would not be like SARS. It would not be like MERS. It would not be like the 1918 influenza pandemic. It was not the plague.

Those predictions, as it turned out, were half-right. COVID-19 was finally named on February 11, a simple abbreviation of "coronavirus disease 2019." The day after, China's death toll surpassed 1,100, and more than 46,000 cases were confirmed. Outside of the epicentre, twenty-four countries were also reporting cases. Then, on Valentine's Day, the virus killed an eighty-year-old tourist in Paris. Cases in South Korea surged, all linked back to one church and one woman. Then, Italy. Haunting images emerged of iconic, seemingly never-empty streets, now policed and abandoned; painfully sparse sick bays housed rows of masked, frail bodies; agonized doctors in robin-blue protective gear told of rationing vital equipment, choosing who would live and die. For healthcare workers in

Canada, it became another signal that perhaps we would not escape whatever hell was emerging, after all. For many others outside the field, however, the story remained fuzzy, distant— a ship looming on the horizon. That changed on March 11, 2020, when, roughly one hundred days after the first person presented with symptoms in Wuhan, the WHO named COVID-19 a global pandemic.

"WHO has been assessing this outbreak around the clock and we are deeply concerned both by the alarming levels of spread and severity, and by the alarming levels of inaction," said the organization's director-general, Tedros Adhanom Ghebreyesus, at a media conference. At the time of his announcement, there were more than 118,000 cases in 114 countries, and nearly 4,300 people had died. "We have never before seen a pandemic sparked by a coronavirus," he added. "And we have never before seen a pandemic that can be controlled."

When I heard the news, I was in my office at Yonge and Bloor streets, one of the busiest intersections in Toronto, where I work as the deputy editor of *Reader's Digest Canada*. I headed home that night on my usual sardine-tin subway car, stopping at a big box near my apartment for groceries. As I pondered yogourt flavours, another customer, a woman wearing a mask, marvelled at the lack of toilet paper, Lysol, pasta, canned anything. I don't know if she was talking to me, or to no one, but I smiled and said something inane like, "Isn't it wild?" We both seemed shell-shocked. I saw her again at the checkout, apologetically sanitizing the conveyer belt. Behind us, a couple had a cart piled high and clinking. The next morning, I looked out from my building's window, onto another normally busy intersection, and for the first time in the two years I'd lived there, saw no cars. It stayed apocalyptically calm for hours, days, weeks. At night, under a newly pinprick sky, I'd watch busses rattle up and down the street, empty.

As stay-at-home orders were issued across North America in early March, it became clear that the story of the pandemic would be different for women—that, in many ways, the story of the pandemic *was* the story of women. In Canada, women comprise 81 per cent of healthcare workers. Notably, they make up the vast majority of nurses, social workers, and personal support workers (PSWs). Beyond the healthcare front line, the *New York Times* estimated that one in three jobs held by women had been designated as essential during nationwide shutdowns, and that racialized women, specifically, held more essential jobs than anybody else. Throughout the pandemic, these women were tasked with keeping our bodies and minds healthy, with keeping us fed, with keeping our hospitals and public spaces clean, with helping the most vulnerable among us, and with being near our bedsides when we died. They led us through, even as they lost the most, and the harsh, uncomfortable truth is that sometimes they led us simply because they couldn't afford to lose more.

To compound all of this, at the same time they were performing these essential jobs, many women abruptly became responsible for home-schooling their kids, juggling their children's needs with their own, often without support. Single and low-income mothers scrambled to buy diapers, to figure out child care, to keep scraping by. Still more women lost their income, accounting for 62 per cent of the job losses between late February and March, and for 50 per cent more vanished work hours than men. Women between the ages of twenty-five and fifty-four, in particular, lost more than two times the jobs that men did. Economists began calling the chilling economic nosedive in North America the "she-cession," noting that for the first time in history, women were more affected by mass job losses than men. And, as COVID-19 swept through long-term care (LTC) homes in Canada at twice the rate of other developed countries, we also became one of the only places in the world where more women than men were getting sick and dying. Many people's worlds were getting smaller, scarier, more uncertain, but it was arguably women who felt this most keenly—women who balanced barefoot on the razor's edge.

But it was also women who, amid the horror and disaster, gave us hope, leadership, and resilience. Across Canada, when we were at our most isolated, women brought us together. On Facebook, two Toronto women, Mita Hans and Valentina Harper, decided to reach out to their neighbours with a modest question: How can we help? The resulting mutual aid group—who, in a refusal to give in to doomsday fearmongers, cheekily named themselves "Caremongers"—quickly became a worldwide movement. Within a month, similar groups had formed across the United Kingdom, Malaysia, India, Pakistan, and the United States, all with the intent of ensuring their community's most vulnerable were not, once again, forgotten. Women banded together to organize mask-making drives, stitching and distributing over 220,000 free coverings through the grassroots group Canada Sews. Elsewhere, women offered free emergency therapy services to frontline workers and organized funding drives to pay people's bills when their Canada Emergency Response Benefit didn't arrive fast enough. In Nova Scotia, Black women lobbied for COVID-19 testing sites in historically overlooked and underserviced neighbourhoods. In every city and town, women were determined to bring out the best in us, even when we were told to expect the worst. People gave millions of dollars, gave time, gave themselves.

"It was such a huge undertaking," said Lee-Anne Moore-Thibert, who founded Canada Sews. "It was such a huge show of Canadian spirit." When she started the group on March 22, she named it Durham Sews, thinking she'd just make a few masks with a few friends for Oshawa, Ontario, and, maybe, the surrounding region. Within twenty-four hours, she had received eight hundred requests and more than three hundred people had joined her sewing army. Watching the numbers climb, she remembers joking with her husband, like, "Ha-ha-ha, let's see if we can hit fifty thousand masks." It was the most far-fetched number she could think of—so distant and so big it didn't even really seem like a goal. But within a few days, the group had grown large enough that she'd renamed it Ontario Sews. Within a week, it became Canada Sews. There were so many requests, and so many volunteers to coordinate, that Moore-Thibert, who is also a managing partner at a paralegal firm, an at-home caregiver for her mother-in-law, and had recently given birth to her first child, was working twenty-two hours every day. She'd wake up at 5 a.m. to nurse her daughter, answer requests, and coordinate volunteers. And, on April 30, when the organization hit that previously unimaginable number of fifty thousand mask deliveries, she broke down and cried. It felt like every hour was filled with fear about the future, but at least she could say that, when it seemed like the world was ending, she did one thing that helped people.

Beyond these everyday small acts of leadership, were the big, life-or-death ones. I have never seen so many women leaders—or their compassion, vulnerability, and humanity— so widely celebrated. In Vancouver's Gastown, artists painted colourful, calm-faced murals of Dr. Theresa Tam and Dr. Bonnie Henry. Others emblazoned the likenesses of the country's many women public health officers on T-shirts, coffee mugs, posters, and pins, usually donating proceeds to various foodbanks and charities. In Alberta, where Deena Hinshaw is the chief medical officer of health, in just six days, one woman sold over 750 shirts that read "What Would Dr. Hinshaw Do?," giving all $20,023 in sales to the province's foodbanks. B.C.'s Henry, easily the most popular of the bunch, even got her own fan club and a namesake pink-and-plum John Fluevog shoe. In June, the *New York Times* ran a profile of her under the headline "The Top Doctor Who Aced the Coronavirus Test." Looking warily toward the failed leadership to the south during the first wave, observers praised the way Canada's majority-women medical leadership navigated one of the worst crises in modern history. Henry's practical advice mantra resonated and reverberated, becoming both a balm and a gospel: "Be kind, be calm, be safe."

Of course, watching the news in those early weeks, very little felt safe. After Italy shocked the world, harrowing images began to emerge from New York's frontline battle. Photos circulated of overfilled funeral homes and morgues. In one, rows of cardboard boxes arranged in neat columns lined a darkened room, with bold labels reading "head" all pointing in the same direction. In another, an army of refrigerated trucks filled the parking lot of a morgue, providing ready-made extra storage for the too-full funeral homes. Trenches opened on New York's Hart Island, packed with unadorned wood boxes holding the city's unclaimed dead. In Brooklyn, bodies in garish orange bags hemmed hospital hallways and loading bays. Here in Canada, cases cascaded through long-term care facilities. Sophie Grégoire Trudeau tested positive for the virus, and Justin Trudeau, in self-isolation, began giving daily updates from the steps of Rideau Cottage. Canada's borders closed. News headlines and social media feeds flickered rising case counts, deaths, panic, disbelief, misinformation.

Now, people called it the plague—though others called it a hoax.

For those of us not on the front lines, the stretch of hours at home could oscillate between fear and boredom, coping and denial. During the first months of the pandemic, we baked lumpy banana bread and sourdough starters, and binge-watched *Tiger King*. We put together puzzles, made whipped coffee, and wondered why every streaming service wanted us to watch *Contagion*. We shifted our social circles to Zoom, watched our own face freeze in triple chins, said our *I love you*s to foreheads. We walked our dogs and held our breath as we jogged past other people, veering onto empty roads. At night, we could not sleep and we scrolled and clicked, read the terrible news over and over. All of us waited for updates, more information, new ways to be safe. We learned about the pandemic in statistics and covered faces and brief obituaries. But we didn't always hear about the women on the front lines, struggling to keep us healthy, struggling to keep us fed, struggling to keep the country from falling apart. We didn't always have the time, or emotional space, to listen.

Women of the Pandemic is meant to remedy that. While it cannot examine the entirety of the ongoing pandemic, it can endeavour to introduce you to the women who led us through the first year—and who, in doing so, changed the world. This book will tell you who they were, what they feared, and what kept them going in the dark. It will tell you about their hopes for us and themselves, about their triumphs and their terrible losses. It will illuminate what they did, and why they matter, and it will work to keep their generation-defining experiences from being erased—by silence, by inattention, by dismissal. Together, these women's stories capture an extraordinary, unprecedented, life-altering year. Their resilience is inspiring. And the myriad ways in which society failed them are devastating. Women have never before played such a vital, essential role in a global crisis, and they've never been the ones who suffered the most. The societal progress of the past two centuries has put them at the messy, murky front. We didn't always take care of them. Now, as we exit the first year of the pandemic, we owe it to these women to pay attention, to remember both their victories and their sacrifices.

In the following chapters, you will walk COVID-19 wards alongside emergency room doctors and nurses, hospital cleaners, hospitality workers, PSWs, and infectious disease researchers. You will feel the curved bow of their slumped shoulders and their grief. You will sit next to a trucker on her return from a long-haul delivery from the U.S., burning with fever, delirious and unable to cross the border and go home. You'll attend the funeral of a woman who worked at a meat processing plant with her husband, and who contracted the virus during one of Canada's worst early outbreaks. You will meet grocery store workers with aching feet and pounding heads, full of worry and exhaustion; mothers who juggled impossible task loads, who were pushed out of their jobs, who gave birth during a swirling pandemic; entrepreneurs who balanced their businesses on the brink, who lost livelihoods, who lost dreams; hospital workers who endured racist, anti-Asian slurs while riding the bus, on their way to keep us all safe. You will understand what it is to don layers of personal protective equipment (PPE) before dashing to swab Canada's first COVID-19 patient, kickstarting vital research into the mystery virus. You will feel the twinning determination and loneliness of one of the country's top vaccine researchers as she gets closer and closer to a solution in a lab far from home, not having seen her children in months. And you will slip behind closed doors and witness decisions that saved, and frustrated, the country.

"I would go home to my husband and say, 'You don't understand,'" says Fiorella Talarico, a sixty-year-old hospital cleaner in Ontario's Peel Region, who, during the first wave of the pandemic, primarily worked on the COVID-19 floor. What she meant was: nobody could understand the exact toll of COVID-19 until they had witnessed the front line; until they had seen dozens of intubated patients, eerily empty waiting rooms, void of anxious families and loving visitors, rooms occupied one day and not the next; until they came home, day after day, and burst into tears. Talarico quickly realized people were experiencing the pandemic in separate realities. In one, the virus was distant, still scary but also unlikely—a bogeyman that wrecked economies, vacations, mental health, and social bonds. In another, hers, it was a mind-boggling, untreatable onslaught of death and pain—a fickle Grim Reaper that claimed both the susceptible and previously healthy, unyielding and without reason. *Women of the Pandemic* aims to merge those realities, to bring us closer to one another, and to ground us in our shared humanity: to help us see how, as Talarico put it, "COVID-19 changed all of us."

I'm writing this introduction in July 2020, and I'm still afraid. I'm afraid when I see photos of exuberant crowds of bronzed and burned bodies at the beach, at the park. I understand why they want to hug each other, delight in casual touch, share a beer. I understand and empathize with their need for connection, but I am afraid of their disregard, of their selfishness. I am afraid for the countries that appear to have given up on containing the virus, and I'm afraid for those who are so fatigued with this fight they appear to have forgotten it. I am very afraid of those who believe the virus doesn't exist, that governments played make-believe with a pandemic, that the current worldwide death count of over 161,000 is inconsequential. A couple of weeks ago, on my thirty-sixth birthday, a sixtyish woman in a white sundress and gold jewellery confronted my aunt and me about our masks. It was sweltering out and she asked if we enjoyed wearing them. We carefully told her they were a pain but that they were necessary for everyone's safety. She shook her head at us, the fools, and remarked, "It's all a hoax."

There is a generous reading of such deliberate distortion. That is, in the face of enormous global upheaval and a forever-altered world, perhaps it is human to want to deny. Maybe certain pandemic conspiracy theorists and rule-breakers have something in common that everybody else, however angrily, can understand: an inability to confront the immeasurable loss of COVID-19. It's tempting to pretend nothing has to change; it's daunting to accept there is no firm end date. But to do either is to undercut every death, every sacrifice, every loss, every woman who did her job. In this time of large, unfathomable griefs, I have my own small griefs, too. Like many of us, I haven't seen my family in months. I haven't celebrated over dinner, or toasted a glass. My hair has split ends and I have cried alone, more times than I can count. My boxing club—my place of community, strength, and mental stillness—didn't make it through the pandemic. I have spent the early stages of Toronto's reopening this summer masked and helping to tear down a place that felt like a second home, or sometimes a first. Even as we mourn, though, we reimagine. For now, my club meets in a public park and, spread six feet apart, we punch the air. Next year: who knows? All of us are trying.

It's impossible to guess at the full consequences of COVID-19. University of British Columbia sociology professor Sylvia Fuller said in July of the disproportionate impact of the virus on women, "By this point it's become clear that the pandemic is not the 'great equalizer.'" As much as we pine for, or rush toward, the new normal, the pandemic isn't over. We cannot know how far the ripples will extend, or what else will be redrawn. Surely, we'll see both good and bad changes, resurgent kindness and unaffordable setbacks. Already, we've seen calls for better social supports, health care, and higher pay for essential workers. Already we've seen a widening gender pay gap, an uneven return to work, and an increase in gender-based violence. As we attempt to chart our paths forward, it's important for us to reflect on this exceptional year, to honour it, and to unflinchingly examine its darkest truths. So, yes, let us rebuild with hope and generosity, but first let us pause and pay attention to what this time, and these extraordinary women, have to teach us.

"IT CERTAINLY HASN'T BEEN BORING."

Dr. Vanessa Allen,
Public Health Ontario

One

THE PANDEMIC ARRIVES

For Dr. Samira Mubareka, January 2020 was the taut silence of an oncoming Maritime storm. The Toronto virologist grew up in Saint-Joseph-de-Madawaska, and was used to watching the wide New Brunswick skies darken, rend, still. Then, *plop*— one bell-shaped raindrop, rippling into an echo. Then, a few lazy seconds later, another. A strange stillness before the downpour. This anticipation felt like that, only worse. Much worse. She knew her hospital, Sunnybrook Health Sciences Centre, was equipped to handle a high-consequence pathogen. When Ebola hit in 2015, they screened patients under investigation for the deadly virus. Every year, her team also screens returning travellers with possible symptoms of MERS, a coronavirus with an alarming fatality rate. They were already planning for a what-if pathogen exercise with multiple public health agencies, scheduled for February. Mubareka herself had spent a decade building capacity at the hospital's infectious disease lab, focusing on respiratory illnesses. If any place could be prepared for a new virus outbreak, it was Sunnybrook.

And yet, with each suspected case of the world's new mystery illness, the knots in her stomach pulled tighter. *Is it starting?* Then, one Thursday evening late that month, another drop fell. A fifty-six-year-old man who had been travelling in Wuhan, China, for three months began coughing on his flight home. The next day, he turned feverish, his temperature pitching to 38.6 degrees Celsius. Paramedics arrived in full PPE and hightailed it to Sunnybrook, where receiving nurses waited, safety gear obscuring familiar cheery scrubs. Doctors tested the man for at least seven different viruses, including SARS-CoV-2, which causes COVID-19, then still-unnamed. He wasn't having trouble breathing, but a lung X-ray showed splotches spread like tree roots. Soon, Mubareka got the call: positive. He was Canada's first confirmed novel coronavirus case; his wife soon became the second. Within forty-eight hours, Mubareka's team had secured permission to collect samples from the patient, from his room, and from the air around him. The knot in her gut constricted.

Mubareka donned her N95 mask, gown, gloves, and protective booties. Of all the sites she'd ever visited, this would be the "hottest"—microbiologist parlance for pretty damn bad. It had been barely a month since China had reported its first case, and little was known about how the virus was transmitted, what it did to the body, how contagious it was, or how deadly. To answer those questions, and to have any hope of stopping, treating, or vaccinating it, scientists needed to study it, whatever it was. But to do that, they first needed samples, lots of them. Not knowing where the virus lurked, Mubareka decided to take surface swabs from several high-touch areas, including the washroom, bed railings, and door handles, as well as bioaerosol samples from both near the man's head and around the room. She felt bad shuffling around him, dressed like an astronaut, the two of them silent; he didn't speak English and she didn't speak Chinese. She could tell he was scared. It would have been nice to talk while she worked, to reassure him as she was swiping and bagging, setting cannisters to capture the air.

Somewhere at the back of her mind, worry hummed. She wondered what would happen if there were a breach. The virus was—and, for that matter, still is—enigmatic. She had no idea if she would survive it, if her immune system could battle it. This new bug was unlike anything science currently understood. What would happen if a single particle, called a virion, slunk inside her body? She was used to handling human viruses, but only when they were captive and controlled in a flask or cryotube. The patient was in a negative pressure room, which allows air to flow into the room but not to escape it, under strict entry and exit protocols. She knew she was as safe as she could be. But none of those details changed the fact that Mubareka was taking samples from a living, very sick man who was potentially expelling a killer virus with every troubled breath. She worked quickly and efficiently. Within ten minutes, she was out. She stripped her safety gear and, just for good measure, immediately showered. She had secured

Canada's first sample of the virus and jump-started vital research. In response, the knots stitched tighter. Now that the country had its first case, how much worse would it get?

Within days, Sunnybrook admitted another potential SARS-CoV-2 case. Then another. And another—each one a fat raindrop, pinging faster. Mubareka collected sample after sample, eventually hitting ten, twenty, fifty. (By the end of 2020, she would collect thousands.) Her team moved to secure permission to work on the virus in her lab at Sunnybrook. By then, it was nearing the end of February. The virus had finally been named but had not yet been declared a pandemic. Mubareka didn't need the official designation to know now. She felt like she had aged five years; stress had winnowed her body. Guilt pooled as she spent day after day, hour after hour, at the lab. She missed her husband and her two children, ages eight and ten, and felt heartbroken about not being there for them. But at least the knot in her stomach had started to unspool. "As more patients arrived at the hospital," she says, "there was almost this sense of relief." That horrible anticipation, that sense of watching the fraught and roiling sky, was gone. She didn't have to wonder what would happen anymore. The storm was here.

On January 3, the last day of her Christmas vacation, Dr. Vanessa Allen absconded to a nearby café. The chief of microbiology and laboratory science at Public Health Ontario (PHO) wanted to catch up on work before Monday, and she needed somewhere quiet, secluded, and, most importantly, away from her twin three-year-olds to do it. ("I love them," she said, laughing. "But they're little monsters.") She was checking her emails when she saw an alert about the worsening situation in Wuhan. Allen had worked in a hospital during the SARS outbreak, had seen the devastation and disorganization first-hand, and had joined PHO because of the agency's mandate to anticipate and better respond to outbreaks. Launched in 2008, PHO is a direct result, as the organization's first annual report puts it, of "Ontario's wake-up call from a series of outbreaks." Those included SARS, of course, but also Legionnaires' disease and the E. coli outbreak in Walkerton. When Allen joined the organization that same year, the province was in the midst of a listeriosis outbreak linked to contaminated cold cuts from Maple Leaf Foods. It eventually killed more than twenty people. Since then, it had seemed like the province had to contend with a possible outbreak nearly every week. She couldn't exactly say a worldwide pandemic was in her comfort zone, but by 2020 she'd had two decades of experience working with outbreaks. She wasn't about to panic—and besides, nobody had yet guessed how big the outbreak was about to become. There was something about its potential, though, that did make Allen want to move fast. She called her colleagues, and by the end of the day they had a testing algorithm in place should anybody in Ontario turn up with symptoms.

At the time, the full genomic sequence of SARS-CoV-2 didn't even exist. But Allen and her team knew the virus was similar enough to both MERS and SARS for them to make what was, essentially, a very educated scientific guess—one that could give them a jump-start on testing. About a week later, on Saturday, January 11, Chinese health authorities released the full sequence for SARS-CoV-2, confirming its striking similarity to the other coronaviruses (and, in particular, to two unnamed bat-derived coronaviruses). That same weekend, Allen's team completed their first test. The results were negative for the virus, and so too was every other test the team performed over the next week. Their ironically lucky strike-out record didn't stop the team from saying yes to testing every sample sent to the lab. If you were the on-call microbiologist during that time, you were constantly fielding calls, accepting samples. In what turned out to be a controversial decision, Allen decided to test everything she was asked to, no matter how unlikely it was to be SARS-CoV-2. As worry multiplied, she made it clear to anxiety-filled hospitals that she would never refuse a request. "It was a huge debate," she said of the policy. "People were worried we were making more of it than we needed to."

There are countless ways a human body can get sick. Before the microscope was perfected in the 1600s, scientists tended to blame outbreaks on everything from social class to divine punishment to clouds of disease-laden air. To them, the idea that an imperceptible organism could invade a person's body and cause illness or even death would have sounded far more ludicrous than even their most bizarre theories. But the microscope literally opened a rich, new world to discovery—that of germs. Working in Berlin, Robert Koch discovered the first bacterium, *bacillus anthracis*, which causes anthrax, in 1876. In time, bacteria became classified as living, single-celled creatures that can cause deadly infections in their host. Bacteria cells are not so dissimilar to mammalian ones, although they are far more simplistic. Think of an air balloon that contains water, nutrients, and a single molecule of DNA. They can replicate on their own and cause harm by directly killing their human host's cells, or by triggering an immune response so severe it damages a person's body. Bacteria's long-awaited discovery led scientists to finally declare the cause of relatively common diseases such as tuberculosis, cholera, and syphilis. The cause of certain other prevalent and deadly diseases, like smallpox, however, remained a mystery. Scientists took sample after sample, but no bacteria could be found.

Initially, they assumed such diseases must be caused by bacteria that were too tiny to be captured through the microscope. They were half-right. It wasn't until the 1930s, with the invention and development of the more powerful electron microscope, that they were able to finally detect the much smaller microbes. Unlike bacteria, viruses are not cells. They consist of a protein coat, called a capsid, inside which the virus stores its genetic material, which in turn carries the code for making new viruses. Many viruses may be deadly, but they lack one key thing: any of their own biochemical machinery to build more particles. In other words, they can't procreate on their own. Viruses overcome this by invading a host's cells and hijacking their machinery to transform them into virus-making factories. In the process, they usually kill the cell itself, either through nutrient depletion or the creation of a toxic environment. After this, sometimes the cell will burst, sending more virus particles into the body. Today, it's estimated that our immune system goes to war against tens of millions of germs every single day. Of them, viruses are the most ubiquitous: they're at least ten times more common than bacteria, and there are at least a hundred million different types. In fact, they are the most plentiful lifeform on Earth—and, every now and then, a new one comes along.

After completing dozens of tests that identified other viruses and bacteria, Allen received Mubareka's sample. Also a clinician at Sunnybrook, she knew about the patient's symptoms and history, and like Mubareka, she suspected this sample would, finally, be a match. Allen ran the virus test only a few days after her twins' birthday, which was on January 16. After the sample was confirmed positive for SARS-CoV-2, she barely saw her family again for months. Her life became a blur of planning, testing, meeting, and troubleshooting—she was in charge of, or a key voice for, it all. During that time, additional leadership responsibilities were also heaped onto her plate: she became the executive lead for PHO's lab response and served as the inaugural medical director of the provincial diagnostic network housed at Ontario Health. From the beginning, Allen worked seven days a week, often for eighteen hours a day. It wasn't uncommon for her to be booked into a mind-boggling twenty-four meetings in a single day. If women had been historically relegated to the scientific sidelines during past pandemics, then it was clear to Allen things would be different this time. Every gender lined the *Brady Bunch*–style tiles of her virtual meetings, and many of the leaders she dealt with most frequently were women.

When I spoke to Allen shortly after the six-month mark of the pandemic, she had just started taking one day off a week. Like Mubareka, she worried about her singular focus on work and felt guilty about being so unavailable to her family. In trying to explain her new-normal busyness, she picked a random day from her calendar, April 6. On that day, she led discussions on finding better processes around the province's prioritization and allocation of testing swabs; prepped for an urgent meeting with the premier's office; sat in on Ontario's weekly command table gathering, which assembles experts from across the province to discuss their concentrated approach to COVID-19; launched and met with another testing strategy panel to address what she saw as a lack of diversity in voices at the table; and helped plot a way to fix underserviced testing areas in Ontario's north—to name only a few things. An average day might include more, but rarely less. "So," she quipped, "it certainly hasn't been boring."

As the night slipped in, Dr. Alyson Kelvin put down her glass of wine and closed her book. Ready for sleep, she reached to turn off her light and, like so many of us, decided instead to check her email one last time. At 11:59 p.m. on December 30, she had received an alert from the Program for Monitoring Emerging Diseases, or ProMED-mail, a free email service with over eighty thousand subscribers—the same service from which Allen received her January 3 alert. Kelvin, who is a virologist at Dalhousie University and the IWK Health Centre in Halifax, jokingly calls it "a social network for infectious disease researchers." Started in 1994, and run by the International Society for Infectious Diseases, the global listserv has been the first to report on SARS, MERS, Ebola, and Zika outbreaks. Because the open-access service also tracks potential toxins and emerging diseases in animals and plants, however, not every notice is so dire. Kelvin points to one email from Russia about a fungus outbreak in radishes, dryly noting why she doesn't read every alert. But this one—featuring a broken English translation from a Chinese news site, emailed under the subject line "Undiagnosed pneumonia, China"—caught her attention.

ProMED editors warned that the social media chatter surrounding the virus sounded eerily similar to the early reports that swirled around SARS. "Returning to the rumor mill," read the email, archly noting an absence of concrete information, "the discussion of this outbreak involves an 'atypical pneumonia.'" The estimated case count was "apparently" twenty-seven, a rapid-fire, perverse connect-the-dots that happened in a matter of days, weeks at most. Kelvin was alarmed: if so many people were hospitalized, the pathogen must be severe. How many others were sick but not at the hospital? She wasn't ready to wave the pandemic flag, but she did want to know more. Kelvin forwarded the email to her father, David, who is also an infectious-disease researcher at Dalhousie and who had established a lab in the Guangdong province of China in 2003 after the SARS outbreak. His response the next day was brief: "Interesting." And, it was. The word *dangerous* would come later.

Though Kelvin had hoped for more, the new pneumonia-like virus wasn't yet on her father's radar—it was hardly on anyone's radar in Canada during the first party-hangover days of 2020. But Kelvin couldn't let it go, especially as more people were hospitalized. She reasoned that they couldn't all have gone to the wet market in Wuhan and interacted with the same species, even *if* that's where the virus originated. It seemed much more likely that, despite assurances otherwise, the unknown virus could spread through human-to-human contact. If that were true, she worried the global consequences of a spillover could be catastrophic. Her lab at Dalhousie was not equipped to study such deadly pathogens, so she reached out to the University of Saskatchewan's Vaccine and Infectious Disease Organization—International Vaccine Centre. More commonly known as VIDO-InterVac, the sprawling lab is a world leader in vaccine research and development. She asked them, "Do you have the virus? Can you get it?"

The new virus wasn't yet a blaring-red warning for VIDO, either. But Kelvin pushed, and researchers there acquiesced.

Before Canada even had its first case, the lab had their permits in place to work on the virus if—when—it arrived. In the meantime, Kelvin began writing research grants to fund what she saw as the inevitable work she would undertake on SARS-CoV-2. It was mid-January, and she kept having to rewrite the sentence charting the global case count. Every time the numbers went up, she'd reopen the document, delete the number, type in a new one. *January 23: 570. January 30: 7,818. January 31: 9,800.* Delete, replace, delete, replace, do it again. As she wrote, she also planned her trip to VIDO, ticking off each step in the complicated clearing process. Background check, done. Supplies gathered, done. Eventually, the only thing left to do was wait. And then came the call from Public Health Ontario: Sunnybrook had the country's first case, and Mubareka had agreed to share her sample with VIDO. On February 24, Kelvin, her graduate student, Magen Francis, and a technician got on a plane.

If early 2020 felt like a storm to Mubareka, to Kelvin it felt like walking down a long, pitch-dark hallway, the only light shining straight at your feet. You could guess your way forward but never know every direction, what was beyond your own private circle of dusk, or how far you had left to go. It wasn't impossible for her to imagine a pandemic; she knew as she packed her suitcase in February that March would look different. People would not be hollering, shoulder-to-shoulder, in crowded stadiums. They would likely not be jet-setting on spring vacations. But as for how bad it would get, and how far it would spread—she had no idea. The unpredictability terrified her, especially as a mother of two young daughters. Initially, she followed her plan to stay at VIDO for three and a half weeks, studying the virus and beginning work on a vaccine, and to then return home. By that time, the world had plunged into the dark hallway alongside her.

The WHO declared COVID-19 a worldwide pandemic on March 11, not long before Kelvin's flight back to Halifax. She stayed home for a week before hopping back on the plane. "I realized even before I left that I needed to come back," she said. "I needed to continue." So she checked into a hotel with a small kitchenette, hung up her clothes, discovered her favourite takeout. Just four more weeks, she thought. Another month and then she'd have done enough research into how the virus transmitted. She'd have answered her questions about why men seemed so much more susceptible than women to severe disease symptoms and hospitalizations. She'd know the life cycle of the virus, what it did to the body, and when. And in knowing all that, she'd know how to stop it from taking over a body, infecting its cells, waging war at the molecular level. She'd have done enough to help VIDO develop a vaccine. Except COVID-19 proved remarkably elusive, evading answers, patterns, logic. The first month passed. Then, the second. Then another and another and another.

In Canada, there are only a handful of Biosafety Level 3 labs—the classification given to facilities that are equipped to study the world's most deadly pathogens. Normally, they compete: for research grants, funding, prestige—for the ability to say they did something first or published earlier than everyone else. Scientific discoveries are guarded, progress kept secret. If it were another time, or if Mubareka were another type of scientist, she might have decided to keep Canada's first COVID-19 sample to herself. Instead, she gave her blessing for every sample she initially collected to be shipped to VIDO, where, because of Kelvin's early insistence, the lab was already set up to study the virus. When Sunnybrook was ready to begin its own work on the virus in late February, Mubareka made another decision: once her team was successful in isolating SARS-CoV-2, she'd share the virus with any Canadian Level 3 lab that wanted it. Forget competition. If the world were to stand a chance against the swiftly moving pandemic, open science needed to triumph. She wasn't the only one who thought so. Soon, other scientists were repeating her new mantra. "It's better to collaborate than to compete," they said.

But to collaborate on anything, someone first needed to isolate the virus. Having a clean and endless source of SARS-CoV-2 would allow Canadian scientists to decode the virus's genetic material, to infect other cells, and to run infinite test models. Without such a supply, it would be impossible to develop any effective medical countermeasures against COVID-19, including antivirals and vaccines. Isolating the virus would be a tricky task, though, and would involve what Mubareka calls "a little old-school virology." Not only was

SARS-CoV-2 new, but science had only recognized the wider coronavirus family itself in the 1960s—to a collective yawn. Scientists largely ignored the bunch of them for decades (even though two of the forty different types are responsible for between 15 and 30 per cent of "common cold" symptoms). They simply weren't deadly enough to be interesting. That is, until the first SARS-CoV virus emerged in 2003, spreading from a bat to a person to the world, before it largely fizzled out a year later. Even then, when the close biological copy of SARS-CoV-2 struck, many virologists in Canada were still focused on other, more lethal things—Zika, West Nile, HIV. As Mubareka has said, "We are really starting from scratch."

Luckily, a few important traits of SARS-CoV-2 were familiar. Like any other virus, a coronavirus needs a host cell to survive. When an infected person sneezes or coughs, they expel virus-loaded droplets into the air and onto surfaces, giving the virus its chance to propagate. From there, a healthy person may inhale or touch a droplet, ushering the virus into their body and laying out an unintentional welcome mat at their nose and throat. The coronavirus will then hijack the cell's machinery, creating endless doppelgangers, invading and infecting, typically moving further and further into the respiratory system. Within their core, coronaviruses all have a strand of RNA, similar to DNA in that it contains the genetic information of the virus, including what information it needs to replicate—a sort of *Art of War* for disease. A lipid-based barrier encapsulates and protects the RNA genome, and also anchors the structural proteins it needs to keep spreading. (Like most fatty things, that barrier breaks down under soap and water, which is why hand-washing works.) Lastly, the crown-like protrusions, called spike, allow the virus to latch on to the body's cells, cracking their defences like an egg.

The "old-school virology" Mubareka drew from involved using viral culture to support, and spur, that SARS-CoV-2 growth process. Ironically, to reach the end goal of killing the virus, scientists first had to give it life. This type of virology stretches back decades. In 1933, scientists isolated the influenza A virus using ferrets. In this case, the Sunnybrook team decided to try a non-human primate, landing on the kidney cell of an African green monkey. Known as Vero cells, and first derived in 1962 from a dissected monkey in Japan, they are popular among virologists because of their high susceptibility to, well, nearly everything. Along with Arinjay Banerjee, a post-doctoral research fellow at McMaster who bunked in her spare room to save precious commuting time, Mubareka then began the trial-and-error process of cultivating the virus. After deciding on the culture, she gathered viral swabs from COVID-19 patients and, working with the rest of the team, put each infected swab into a viral transport media. From there, Mubareka would give whatever swab she was working with a little shake, causing the virus to glide off, becoming suspended in the medium. Moving carefully, she'd then take the now virus-laden medium and drop it into a tray of small wells, not unlike Jell-O moulds. Next, she'd rock the mixture gently, allowing the virus to rise to the top of the culture cells. "And then it's kind of like waiting for a cake," Mubareka said, laughing—you do nothing for a little bit, but, if you got everything right, the virus will grow.

On the other hand, a lot can go wrong. If you take a sample from a person's nose, for example, you might inadvertently scoop up pesky immune factors, impeding the virus's ability to spawn. Certain bacterial toxins could contaminate your sample. Or, you might have cultivated a different coronavirus entirely. If Mubareka and Banerjee had done any of that, they wouldn't have known right away. A human cell is about 10,000 nanometres; a coronavirus is 90 nanometres, scant billionths of a metre (and, for that matter, also much smaller than any type of bacteria)—meaning that, even when the human eye has help, without an electron microscope, the virus is more or less invisible. Instead, Mubareka had to rely on seeing the damage. The first time they tried to cultivate the virus, the monkey cells looked "unhappy," but the team wasn't convinced it was the destructive work of SARS-CoV-2. So, they decided to try to trick the virus again into doing what it does best: ravaging. And, on the second try, they saw it more clearly. Now, there were holes where the virus had caused cells to disintegrate, called a cytopathic effect—think of it as a punched-out paper snowflake. It was promising, but Mubareka wouldn't be convinced until a molecular test confirmed the virus's full genome sequence. She noted, "I'm very conservative with these things."

Within a week, the test clinched it. Shortly after, photos from an electronic microscope confirmed it again, showing the virus's telltale namesake, the *corona*—Latin for "crown." On March 13, Sunnybrook announced that its lab had isolated the virus. Mubareka kept her promise and shared virus cultures with any Containment Level 3 lab that wanted them, which, as it turned out, was most of them. The day Sunnybrook announced the isolation, Canada recorded forty-two new cases, and it was only three days into the pandemic. The more virus samples researchers could now isolate, the better. A virus isn't stagnant. Over time and across geographies, SARS-CoV-2 would likely mutate and evolve, seeking new ways to survive and always, always replicate. Multiple samples and isolates allowed microbiologists to examine and trace its changing nature as it spread, a relentless wave carried on by crowded cities and global travel, a hyper-connected world.

When Amy Greer received the ProMED warning at the end of 2019, her mind blinked back a decade to the 2009 H1N1 influenza pandemic. At the time of the virus' second wave, she had worked for the federal public health agency, supporting the country's pandemic preparedness and response activities. She remembered building mathematical models, estimating and re-estimating the potential spread of what was commonly called swine flu, after its similarity to influenza viruses found in pigs in North America and Eurasia. Like the strange new coronavirus, the then-new influenza had a unique combination of genes that had never been seen in either humans or animals. The first worldwide case was reported in Mexico on March 18, 2009, and it would go on to kill more than four hundred Canadians. Greer, now a professor at the University of Guelph and a Canada Research Chair in Population Disease Modelling, called a few colleagues whom she worked with on H1N1. She wanted to know if they'd also been following the news out of Wuhan.

"I don't know if I'm being paranoid or not," she told them, laughing, just a little, at the absurdity of what she was about to say. "This might be a complete waste of time." Hesitation. "But maybe we should dust off our pandemic models." Her colleagues agreed, and together they started building the necessary code, hoping they wouldn't have to use it. By late February, Greer started going through her pantry, taking stock. Her husband was startled. "He said, 'Geez, normally you're very laid back,'" she recalled. "'If you're telling me we need a quarantine stockpile, then I'm starting to get worried.'" So was Greer. They tried to think of everything they might need. She quizzed herself: *Do we have batteries for the thermometer? Do we have an extra bottle of children's Advil? If everything shuts down, are we ready?* At work, she asked different questions, formulating distinct scenarios based on the dynamics of the emerging pathogen and then projecting that knowledge forward in time: *If we did nothing to mitigate transmission, what would happen a month from now, two, three? What if we retreated, actually did shut down everything, distanced from each other? What if we all wore masks? What would be necessary to slow down transmission?*

Without strict intervention, many possible outcomes showed the same thing: collapse. Epidemiologists and mathematical modellers were still learning about the biology of the virus, but they did know it appeared to be highly transmissible. In scant weeks, the virus had undulated across the globe, spreading through Italy, Iran, and Brazil. It had skulked aboard a cruise ship anchored on a Japanese shoreline, infecting more than six hundred people—at the time, the largest outbreak outside China. Models from different countries, even using slightly different methods, consistently estimated that 60 to 70 per cent of their populations could become infected if the virus were to spread unchecked, without interception by public health. The numbers felt staggering, unfathomable. The air buzzed with the possibility of mass death. It buzzed with denial. Even Greer and her colleagues couldn't say with certainty what would happen. The new coronavirus was behaving in puzzling ways. Most viruses wreak havoc on the very old and the very young. During the 1918 Spanish flu pandemic, mortality rates were particularly high for children under age five. Children also suffered more during swine flu. But SARS-CoV-2 barely seemed to infect children at all. Many wondered if kids were actually faring better or if they just hadn't had the chance to become infected yet.

As new information trickled through to her via open access research networks, Greer adjusted and updated her models, emailing the findings to her network of government contacts and public health officials. The virus may have been a series of question marks punctuated by even bigger question marks, but she did know that, to slow transmission, people needed to significantly change their day-to-day behaviour. She knew it would be a hard sell. In mid-March, many parts of the country still had zero cases. The virus felt terrifying, but also mythical, a fire-breathing dragon, a Marvel villain, something from *over there*. She worried politicians would be willing to wait until there were more cases, and then it would be too late to put on the brakes. Hospital intensive care units would be overwhelmed. Ventilator capacities would buckle. She was surprised, and relieved, when immediate, aggressive stay-at-home orders were issued. She also knew that, despite hopes at the time, three weeks wouldn't be enough. So, when the *National Post* asked her what it would take to stop thousands of deaths, she answered honestly.

For centuries, the idea of social distancing and mass lockdowns have figured strongly in public health responses to disease outbreak. During the 1918 Spanish flu, which would be deeply mined for lessons in pandemic management in the months ahead, cities all over the world limited public gatherings and adjusted business practices. Some did so drastically; others, less so. New York City merely staggered its business hours, for instance, with the aim of reducing crowds. It also educated city-dwellers on the dangers of coughing and spitting in public. Other cities shut down everything, including schools, libraries, movie theatres, stadiums, and any other places where people gathered in mass numbers. San Francisco and San Diego required anybody who went out in public to wear a gauze mask. But, just like with COVID-19, timing mattered. Cities that waited weeks to implement measures—even those with the strictest rules—suffered high mortality rates. (Philadelphia had one of the highest in the U.S.; it knowingly held a parade after the virus had started infecting the city.) Other places that acted immediately, such as St. Louis, fared better. So too did cities that refused to lift restrictions as the pandemic peaked. Then, just as now, the dissemination of information also mattered. Some media downplayed the pandemic, encouraging a false sense of safety. And, on top of that, wrote Joshua Loomis in *Epidemics: The Impact of Germs and Their Power over Humanity*, politicians worldwide couldn't seem to agree on anything: "This produced unnecessary delays and created confusion in populations who often were getting mixed messages." Sound familiar?

One hundred years later, similar sacrifices would be just as difficult to sell to the public. On March 21, the *National Post* printed an article quoting Greer, who said thirty-two weeks of strict public health measures were needed to prevent Canada, and its healthcare system, from becoming overwhelmed. "The challenge in all of this is it's unprecedented," she said. "We're asking people to do something that is really challenging and we're going to be asking them to do it for a very long time." Many people read this as if Greer, personally, were ordering them into a long lockdown. Within hours, she began to get a "boatload" of hate emails. Even family and friends began to reach out, enraged, telling her the virus was a conspiracy, the measures overkill. Strangers told her she was ruining their child's high school graduation, that she'd ended prom, bungled family vacations. Greer was perplexed. In her mind, the message was simple: We need to think about how we're going to keep people safe, or else. In a way, the hateful emails weren't entirely wrong. For people to live and for our healthcare system to survive, graduations and proms would need to be cancelled. Still, while the unexpected onslaught exhausted her, Greer didn't feel bad about sharing data that supported long periods of public health measures, such as physical distancing and mask-wearing. As the country retreated inside, she thought, *It's better than killing your grandparents.*

For centuries, disease has directed—and interrupted—the course of human history. In 430 BCE, during the Peloponnesian War, what is now thought to be typhoid fever passed through Libya, Ethiopia, and Egypt, eventually doing what the Spartans could not: infiltrating Athens. Two-thirds of the population died and, eventually, Athens fell. Centuries later, smallpox claimed Roman Emperor Marcus Aurelius. A century after that, a plague caused an under-attack Britain to seek help from the Saxons against the Picts and the Scots; the Saxons soon controlled the island. Then came the bacterium *Yersinia pestis*—the bubonic plague. In 541, when it first appeared, Romans called it the Justinian plague, after the leader who had attempted, and was to some extent succeeding at, the revival of the once-great empire. It advanced on the world, breaking out again and again until finally fizzling out in 750 CE. By then, it had caused the deaths of some fifty million people, or over one-quarter of the population, thus sparking the apocalyptic atmosphere that fuelled the rise of both Christianity and Islam.

It returned again in 1347, grinding the war between France and England to a halt and decimating the Vikings. The Black Death killed roughly two hundred million people this time, more than half the world's population. It also created a labour shortage and gave peasants the leverage to end feudalism. After that, viruses entered the killing fields in a big way. The spread of smallpox first wiped out the Aztecs and continued on to kill about 90 per cent of North America's Indigenous populations. Smallpox, or the "speckled monster," both facilitated colonialism and decimated a way of life—likely deliberately. Next came cholera, more bubonic plague, the measles, yellow fever, the flu, each toppling armies, governments, empires, and sometimes helping to create new ones. But perhaps no viral outbreak is as relevant today, at least in the wider public mind, as the 1918 H1N1 flu pandemic. It killed fifty million people and prevented the Americans from striking German reparations from the Treaty of Versailles, arguably paving the way for the Second World War. On a more positive note, it also forced massive, long-lasting healthcare reform. As *Pale Rider* author Laura Spinney wrote in her book about the virus, "The Spanish flu resculpted human populations."

The same could be said of polio and HIV. It shouldn't surprise us that, in particular, many of these viruses have proven difficult to eradicate. Some still don't have vaccines. There are many reasons for this, but at least one is that viruses are survivors. Mubareka calls them the "apex adaptors." They have proliferated in impossible places, such as polar ice caps, salt marshes, and acid lakes. It's what first drew her to the infectious diseases field: the unpredictable interconnectedness of it all. Human behaviour and advancement, especially travel, has allowed for sickness that might once have been contained to go anywhere, everywhere. Viruses can't move on their own; they need to hitch a ride on us. Humans, in turn, created unfettered access to, well, everything, and now it's spilling over, which makes the work Mubareka does in her Toronto lab relevant on a global scale. But it's more than that. Only a small percentage of viruses borne by animals will successfully infect a person or an entire population, creating what's called a zoonosis. Some don't evolve enough to overwhelm human cells; others don't achieve high human transmission. As the virus attempts to win, it will make little adaptations here and there, mindlessly working to change its entire story. Mubareka finds it all fascinating. "A couple of amino acids and here we are," she said. "A tiny little molecular machine has effectively brought the world to its knees."

"WE'RE HELPING OUR CANADIAN FAMILY THROUGH THIS PANDEMIC, BUT WE DON'T WANT TO GO HOME SICK."

Pramie Ramroop,
meat processing plant employee

Two

FEEDING A COUNTRY

Nicole Folz didn't dare go home in March 2020. Her mom had diabetes and her dad was older, edging the high-risk line of COVID-19. She didn't want to give the virus to her sister or young niece either. So, even though she felt fine and didn't know a single person who was sick, the twenty-six-year-old did what many other long-haul truckers were doing. Whenever she got back from a trip, she steered her red-and-white Freightliner Cascadia into the company's yard, parked the truck, and called it home sweet home. The lot in Guelph, Ontario, was three hours away from her actual home in Bancroft. It could have been worse. As a trucker, Folz was used to the isolation. If anyone could endure the loneliness, she figured, it was someone like her—a person drawn to long stretches of solitary driving, criss-crossing Canada and the U.S., wanderlust in her bones. Even before she became a trucker in February 2019, she used to get in her Jimmy, drive until she felt like stopping, and spend the night tucked across the seats in a grocery store parking lot. Still, it *was* lonely. She had also refused to see friends she'd made in the area; with all the travel she did and all the people she saw, it was just too risky. "It was kind of like I had the cooties," she said, laughing.

Folz loves her job. While she jokes that she has her "womanly things to keep up with," like getting her nails and lashes done, she's always wanted to work in a traditionally male-dominated field. One of her first gigs was at a lumberyard. She went to college to learn construction drilling and blasting. She likes physical labour, likes knowing that, when a task is done, she did it justice. Plus, when you get right down to it, what she also likes is "making a man's wage." Even in such fields, though, things aren't always so clear-cut. After college, she was working road construction when she found out a kid with zero experience and who was still in high school was paid more than her. It felt like a slap in the face. The discovery helped push her into pursuing the job she really wanted. With the help of a government grant, she signed up for the required training to get the licence she viewed as freedom. She was one of the few people in her class to pass on her first try. Folz has since hauled supplies all over North America, from her Ontario headquarters to Iowa to Louisiana to Georgia.

It was after a pickup in Chicago to get medical supplies, including gloves, masks, gowns, and hand sanitizer, that Folz started to feel unwell. She continued to drive down to South Carolina, playing a denial game the whole time. *It's probably just a cold*, she told herself. It was April 7. Chicago had been in the news as an emerging COVID-19 hotspot, and Folz, who listened to the news sometimes as she drove, knew it. Even as she tried to tell herself not to worry, that thought stuck in her head. Then again, she was only tired and a bit foggy; it could just be a cold. She reassured herself over and over and over. But she wasn't about to gamble with someone else's health. She constantly sanitized her hands and everything she touched, and wore a face mask and gloves when she did the next delivery. Pretty soon, her throat felt like a thousand bees had swarmed it. Raw and sore, she started coughing. After she walked into a building, it felt like she had run a mile to get there. She was hot, too, burning up—then again, she was in South Carolina, where it was already creeping up to 30 degrees Celsius. Maybe she wasn't used to the heat. Folz didn't have a thermometer in her truck, but she knew she needed to get one and take her temperature.

In the meantime, she called her dispatcher and said, "I think I have COVID-19." It was the early afternoon, and Folz was at least a fourteen-hour drive away from her truckyard. Fatigue anchored her limbs; she needed to go back. She also needed sleep, and maybe a hospital. Instead, she had to stay the night and reload the next day. Often when she has a layover, Folz will style her hair, get dressed up, and spend a night on the town. Now, she parked her truck and curled up in the bed located behind her seat. She drifted in and out—strange, fevered dreams hunting peacefulness, rest. In the morning, she bought a thermometer. Her fever had hit 39.3 degrees Celsius. She drove through it, because what else could she do? She couldn't abandon her truck. She couldn't abandon her load. She couldn't check into a hotel and spread the virus there, even if there were room to park the Freightliner. At her stop in South Carolina, she stayed inside the cab until everybody else was gone. "Don't touch anything," she told them. "I'm sick." She felt like hell.

Clutching her pink steering wheel, she felt every hour of driving as if it were six. She usually relished the open expanse of road. Now, she thought it would never end. At every rest stop, she looked at the bed behind her and cried. She'd never longed for anything so badly in her life, but it would only slow her down—and in the middle of nowhere, fever climbing. So she refused to sleep, and the closer she got to the Canada–U.S. border, the more she wondered what she should do. Could she cross? How? Where should she go once she did? How would she get there? She called her parents, who were terrified for her. And she called every public health agency she could think of, more than once, pausing every few words to gulp in air. "What protocols have been put in place?" she asked. "What's the procedure here?" Nobody seemed to know. *Somebody must*, she thought. There were hundreds of truckers on the road, delivering food and essential supplies. Surely, there had to be a plan if they got sick. The federal and provincial governments wouldn't just abandon them.

But when Folz finally arrived at the border on Good Friday, the best option she had was a kind nurse who, during one of her numerous calls to Canadian public health agencies, had offered to let her stay in her backyard.

———

Natasha Grey has worked as a cashier in the same Toronto grocery store since she was eighteen. She can still tell you the day she started: December 23, 1998. Grey grew up in Malvern, the neighbourhood where the store is located, and even after she got married, moved to nearby Pickering, and began to work full-time at CIBC, she never quit. She stays, quite simply, because she cares about her community; good food is at the centre of everything. Plus, her parents and her sister still live in the vibrant neighbourhood, tucked into the northeast corner of the city, bordering Highway 401 and the Toronto Zoo. If you were to stroll along a tree-studded street there, or peruse a low-slung strip mall, you might hear a chorus of Urdu, Tamil, English, Cantonese, and Tagalog. Many of the customers at Grey's big box store are regulars, people who've offered her a kind smile for years, who've watched her become an adult, who always ask after her family. As March bred panic about the pandemic, Grey bought masks, gloves, and Lysol wipes, but she still stayed. She wanted to help her co-workers and the customers she cared about. "At the end of the day," she said, "it all falls back into one thing. We need the grocery store to be open."

Once CIBC allowed her to work from home on her own time, Grey moved her grocery store shifts to early in the morning. Six days a week, she arrived at the store before sunrise and drove home just after lunch. Then, she'd quickly eat a meal and work her second job until 11 p.m., get up exhausted, and do it all over again. She didn't even have time to watch the weather forecast on TV. At her store, all nine lanes were open and the stream of customers was relentless. In the beginning, before the store taped arrows and queues, the lines stretched out through the aisles and around the building's interior. Tensions ran higher than people's fear-built mountains of toilet paper, cleaning products, and canned goods. Grey saw gratitude, but she also witnessed angry jostling, fist fights, and a whole lot of yelling. People bristled at the idea of social distancing. Sometimes, when Grey ventured into the aisles, marvelling at how the store looked like it had been robbed, a customer would tap her on the shoulder: "Excuse me." Grey would take two steps back and warmly ask how she could help. Some customers didn't like that either. They'd bark, "I don't have COVID!" But she couldn't know that. Anybody could have it.

In spring 2020, for Canadians, the grocery store became both a symbol and the real-life pinpoint of our pandemic anxiety. Fear, cruelty, humanity, kindness, impatience, anger— every emotion of the unknown converged as we wondered how long this would last, if we would go without. The uncertainty created its own sort of virus, catching and spreading. We turned into zombies, ravenous, unreasonable, all buying unearthly amounts of tuna. We turned bitter. The grocery store was the only place many of us could go, and it was so different and so out of our control that we hated it. We hated waiting in line, we hated wearing masks, we hated how crushing it was to buy a singular box of pasta when suddenly you absolutely needed two. Even Grey, who felt nervous watching people hoard, started to buy more food than she could eat. Her sister would see her dump rattling boxes of macaroni-and-cheese into a cart and give her a Look. "Don't worry," her sister tried to soothe. "Everything will be okay." But in those early weeks, Grey wasn't so sure. Nothing was in stock at any of the other grocery stores she visited either. She even checked Walmart, a place she doesn't like because it isn't unionized, and it was empty, too. Every morning, she'd wake up and pray, "God, help me today—and always."

She tried to focus on the good moments: the regulars who, after the store put up Plexiglass barriers to protect workers, gave her "air hugs"; a disabled woman who thanked Grey sincerely and profusely after she helped pack her bags, even though to do so was against store policy; another woman who was similarly grateful after Grey gave her a Lysol wipe—that's it, just a Lysol wipe, more precious than gold; her colleagues who joked around and tried to make things seem normal even when nothing was. Some days were harder than others. On one of the hardest, Grey's husband had come to pick her up from work. She was leaving the store when she heard an ear-splitting *BAM!* She turned and saw two men fighting over the last roll of toilet paper. Grey ran over, flabbergasted. If you'd told her in January that only two months later she'd be breaking up a fist fight over Royale or Charmin, she would have laughed. "It's like the pandemic turned certain people into monsters," she said. And every day, there she was: at the gate, her only weapons a kind word, good service, and a smile that nobody could see behind her mask.

Collectively, we spent millions of dollars more on groceries than we usually do in March and April, driven by a mixture of scarcity fear, a dash of boredom, and, understandably, a mass yearning for salt, fat, and sugar. Stress-baking alone drove flour sales up 200 per cent. Workers in the 1300s used their sudden power advantage during the Black Death to end medieval serfdom. With so much of the population cleaved, there were not enough peasants to work the land, and serfs gained unexpected bargaining room. Where they were once legally bound to work the fields with little reward, they now persuaded lords to let them rent plots, with a chance to turn their own profit. It was either that or let the fields rot. These ambitious farmers ushered in an era of better treatment, a fledgling middle class, and a new economic model—a turning point now referred to as the birth of agrarian capitalism. While it seems unlikely that today's essential workers were thinking of the centuries-gone serf system in March and April 2020, their position is remarkably comparable. Many are underpaid and undervalued. In particular, those who work in non-unionized grocery stores, processing plants, distribution centres, farms, and factories often have little job security and therefore scant ability to speak up about mistreatment or unfair practices. And yet, like the lords and ladies of old, the millionaires and billionaires who employ them are arguably raking it in.

As we descended upon grocery stores across the country, COVID-19 handed workers on the front lines of the food and packaging industries their own bleakly fortuitous bargaining chip. Everybody needed them to work. As both customer numbers and COVID-19 case counts surged, thousands of essential workers were unable to stay at home, safely cocooned in a virus-free environment. As a should-be-predictable consequence, many got sick. Some died. Each punch of the clock was a possible death knell, for themselves and their families. Many of them couldn't afford to quit their newly dangerous jobs; some did anyway. As one union president put it, "Who in their right mind would risk contracting COVID . . . for $11.32 an hour?" Companies scrambled to hire new workers and keep the ones they still had. Those who stayed were able to use their newfound "hero" status to rightfully push for hazard pay. Bowing to public pressure, most grocery store chains, including Loblaws, Sobeys, and Metro, as well as some processing plants, such as Maple Leaf Foods, tacked on an extra two dollars to employees' hourly wages. Michael Medline, CEO of Empire, which owns Sobeys, IGA, and Safeway, crowed in late March that such raises, along with other support programs, were "simply the right things to do."

And they were. The pandemic created a new class of frontline workers, expanding the conventional definition of emergency care to people who were never trained for it—people who, quite frankly, had never signed up for it and weren't being compensated for it. Some got relatively lucky, like Grey—despite the extraordinary stress of the job, she said both her union and her employer supported workers. Or, at least they supported them the best they could. Others didn't. It wasn't just that workers were getting sick, although many did; by early May, Loblaws had reported more than 130 cases across its stores, and other large chains reported similar numbers. It was the stress. The knowing that any customer could have the virus, could pass it to you, and leave you to pass it on to everyone you love. It was watching customers hem and haw over whether to get zesty Doritos or cool ranch. Knowing that you were there risking your life every day, working longer hours, being yelled at, and receiving what felt like the world's frustration piled on your shoulders, all so people could get a bag of Oreos. Then you'd hear about the Oshawa department manager who died, the Vaughan distribution centre worker, the Walmart employee. How could you not be afraid? "It takes the energy right out of you," said one Toronto woman, a manager who works at two stores owned by the same chain. "You put all the strength that you have to make it through the day, to be able to do your job, to execute your daily functions. And by the time you get home, you've just got nothing in the tank."

The "right thing" lasted until June. Loblaws, which said it had spent $180 million on extra wages, clawed back its pandemic pay first, then sent its rivals a so-called courtesy email informing them of this step. Everyone else followed. Perhaps unsurprisingly, the move was a bitter pill for many essential workers. One Hamilton, Ontario, grocery store baker who spoke out explained that the wage hike had allowed her to put away savings for the first time since she'd been off maternity leave. Plus, the pandemic, clearly, was still happening. "We're being called essential workers," she said. "Well, you can't take away essential." As cities and other jurisdictions passed mandatory mask bylaws, many workers experienced daily verbal, and even physical, harassment. Videos of hyper-privileged customers berating workers who had politely asked them to wear a mask went viral. Speaking at the time, Medline echoed his earlier language, albeit in a considerably less rah-rah moment: "Should this terrible virus rear its ugly head to the degree that . . . we experienced in March and April, we will put hero pay back into our company stores in those regions or cities," he said. "That would be the right thing to do." (And, in late November 2020, Sobeys did reinstate some form of "hero pay" in three of Canada's hardest-hit regions: Winnipeg, Toronto, and Peel.)

In response to the cuts, senior executives from three major chains were called to speak before a parliamentary committee, their testimony timed like snug dominoes, but little came of it. In late August, eleven Loblaw-owned grocery stores in Newfoundland went on strike over the pandemic-pay cut. That same week, a Loblaws distribution centre in Surrey, B.C., announced a new outbreak. So much for The Birth of Fair Wages.

In many cases, the pandemic flipped the traditional script, putting women on the front lines. A significant number of workers who briefly gained higher (but not high) "hero" wages are women, many of them women of colour. A lot of them are new Canadians, mothers, recent students, seniors: economically vulnerable populations scraping by. They are the people we thanked with colourful, bold signs, staked in lawns and taped in windows. Children wrote pastel tributes to them in sidewalk chalk. We drew hearts and grocery carts and we drew women on signs, happy and uniform. Perhaps you thought of them gratefully when you got home and plopped three browning bananas into a bowl. Or maybe you realized, as you pulled your lumpy bread from the oven, that you could have been nicer when you paid for your flour, yeast, or butter. Maybe you thought, "Thank goodness I only have to do this once a week," as you made it to the front of the winding line, nodded to the security guard, and walked through the automatic doors. Maybe you were one of these workers, just trying to make it through the day before you made it home with your own hard-earned bags of sugar and chocolate, chips and cheese. Maybe, regrettably, you didn't think much about these workers at all. Certainly, there were some people in this comfort-food chain that we didn't see, that we never see—even before the pandemic. Much of the country's mass-produced food system relies on certain invisible workers staying invisible. It took longer for us to thank them, if we did at all.

Pramie Ramroop went to work one morning in March and kept going until July. Seven days a week, she'd arrive early for her 4:55 a.m. shift at a food processing plant in Mississauga. She needed time to don her arsenal of protective gear and get her temperature checked. Ramroop has been an employee at the plant for over two decades. When she was hired, she worked the line for three years, packaging precooked chicken and sauces in box after box. Eventually, she worked her way up to the position of packaging lead hand, what might be called an assistant supervisor. She watches the line run. If there's a breakdown, she figures out how to fix it. She knows every single job required to keep the plant running, and she knows how to do all of them. She's also the person whom many workers come to if they have a question or a complaint, or if they need to share their feelings. And how they were feeling in March and April was scared. Ramroop was also scared. The plant had told workers early on that there would be no days off unless they had a doctor's note—demand for prepackaged, frozen food was through the roof. "We're helping our Canadian family through this pandemic," Ramroop said, explaining the duelling emotions many workers felt. "But we don't want to go home sick."

Even before the pandemic, Ramroop's workplace followed strict safety precautions. Where COVID thrives, so too can nasty, gut-churning bacteria like listeria and salmonella. Anybody entering the plant's ready-to-eat area already had to wear a face covering, hairnet, helmet, protective sleeves, gloves, an apron, and water boots. To get inside, you walk through a sanitizer that sprays white foam on your feet—imagine a car wash for humans, except the effect is more like the fog that eddies the ground at a rock concert. Once you're there, handling all manners of precooked chicken, you're so swathed in protective gear only your eyes show. COVID-19 added face shields, better masks, and extra sanitization. People distanced on the line and started tapping their feet together like Fred Astaire or Gene Kelly to say hello, forgoing hugs. When one person tested positive for the virus, everyone watched, aghast, as the story made the local TV news. Ramroop was just as shaken as everyone else. "Oh my God," employees exclaimed in the lunchroom, on the line, as they passed each other on the floor. "Oh my God, are we going to get it, too?" An entire production line closed so everyone could get tested. The company put more Plexiglass barriers up. Co-workers were forbidden to sit next to each other in the lunchroom. Cleaners regularly sprayed tables, doorknobs, washrooms—everything.

Only one other person at that time at the plant got sick, but it didn't make Ramroop any less nervous. Most of her family were essential workers. Her husband had a job at another food processing plant, one that was much slower to take extra precautions than hers. At the beginning of the pandemic, she drove him to Costco, stockpiled disposable masks, and forced him to wear them. Her son is a paramedic who worked some of the hardest-hit regions of Ontario. She didn't see him for months, but sometimes he would drive by her home in Brampton and they would both wave hello. Her daughter, who lives with Ramroop and her husband, stayed working, thankfully from home. Every day after work, Ramroop bolts straight to the shower. She leaves her boots in the garage, dipped in a bucket of homemade cleaner, sanitizes all the

mats, and after she gets out of the shower everything is sanitized: her lunch bag, those boots, everything she touched.
Every two weeks, someone goes to the grocery store and she'll
sanitize whatever bounty they return with, too. Her son,
who didn't want Ramroop leaving the house more than she
had to, dropped off supplies once. She washed those as well.
Whenever someone stuck flyers in her door, she'd wipe the
doorknobs clean.

Throughout it all, her son helped keep her going, encouraging her to relax. Every day he called to remind her to lie
down and nap. "You're working seven days a week," he'd tell
her. "The time you wake up isn't normal. You're going to get
drained." She was too worried about catching the virus to risk
walking through her neighbourhood, so when the weather
became nicer he coaxed her to spend time in the backyard—
told her to take her vitamins, try some yoga. Day in and out,
he kept her spirits up. Not that Ramroop ever resented the
dogged pace at work. She knew that frozen food might be the
easiest way to put dinner on the table during the toughest
months of the lockdown. People had to work and people were
out of work, and both sets of people had children to feed. She
doesn't even really resent that her two-dollar-an-hour pandemic pay boost lasted only a month, not nearly as long as the
period of intense overtime. What she does wish is that people
like her, those who work behind the scenes, were more publicly acknowledged as essential workers. If not for farmers
and food processing plants, how would all that food even

make it to the grocery stores? "The people who put food on the table," she said. "They didn't get no recognition."

Or if they did, she added, it was because they had died.

The wind whips against Nga Nguyen's grey cargo pants, pleating them haphazardly. It's the first Monday in May, a few hours after the Cargill meat packing plant in nearby High River reopened, and exactly two weeks after Nguyen's wife, Bui Hiep, died after contracting COVID-19 while working there. Nguyen is standing on the green-and-beige grass of Forest Lawn High School, near their Calgary home—now his alone. Through an interpreter, he is trying to explain how he is feeling, but he can't because, really, he isn't feeling anything at all. He's numb. Hiep had worked at the plant since 1996, nimbly picking bones out of beef destined to become hamburger meat. She started to feel ill on Thursday, April 16, but finished her eight-hour shift, sitting on cold metal as an industrial fan blew frigid air at her back. The sixty-seven-year-old was charming and friendly at work, doling out candy to co-workers, and, as one put it, "always winning for 'never absent employee.'" They were probably surprised when Hiep called in sick on Friday with what she thought was the flu. The next day, an ambulance rushed her to the hospital. The day after that, she was gone; Nguyen didn't even have a chance to say goodbye. Now, Nguyen was alone on the grass, in front of a condolence fruit basket and a white banner with orange hearts, attempting to put words to a constellation of grief. "I want to find a way to join my wife," he told the crowd gathered at the memorial service. "I just want to end my life."

Nguyen and Hiep had escaped Vietnam on the same boat after the war. They landed at the same refugee camp, fell in love, and were only briefly separated when Hiep immigrated first to Canada. A year later, in 1993, Nguyen was able to follow and the two were reunited and married. They had a happy, full life, but no children. Nguyen confessed through his interpreter that he had worried about his wife dying and leaving him alone. Now that it had happened, well—the interpreter trailed off as Nguyen did, ending with a plaintive shrug, palms to the sky. The memorial, organized by Action Dignity, a community-based non-profit that supports and advocates for the city's ethno-cultural groups, was in actual effect more of a press conference. For both Action Dignity and Nguyen, the event became a way to immortalize Hiep into more than "the Vietnamese worker who died at Cargill." By then, the plant had laid a notorious claim to the worst workplace outbreak in North America. Almost half of the plant's 2,000 workers had tested positive for COVID-19, and another 609 cases in Alberta had been linked to Cargill employees. At least three, including Hiep, would die. The explanation for this disastrous record was both terrible and simple: Cargill hadn't done enough to protect its workers.

As Edmonton's Poet Laureate, Nisha Patel, wrote in a lengthy, rage-fuelled poem named for Hiep: "how essential the temporary have become, how foreign the ghosts will be when all that's left are the ones that started it, I didn't believe in revenge until I learnt that only managers got the masks." Later media investigations showed that, indeed, Cargill did not widely supply masks to workers in March. Nor did it initially make other changes that might have helped, like installing plastic shields or applying distancing rules. The plant disassembled 4,500 cows per day, all along tightly packed lines, and introducing such measures would have presumably ground down productivity. Some workers did what Ramroop had for her husband: they bought their own masks. Often, they reused them, sometimes for weeks. Other workers tied bandanas over their mouths like cartoon bandits. Not every worker wore protection; Cargill didn't require it, and as of March, the public hadn't widely adopted masks either. A *Globe and Mail* report revealed that many workers felt pressured to come to work, even when they were sick. Multiple employees told the *Globe* they were cleared to return despite symptoms, unfinished self-isolation periods, recent international travel, and—most maddening of all—positive COVID-19 test results. What's more, Cargill released its info bulletins to employees only in English, further sowing confusion at a plant where many employees are temporary foreign workers and new Canadians. Even if what they were reading would have made sense to employees, it's likely many would not have been able to understand it.

As COVID-19 case counts climbed too high to pretend the situation was business as usual, Cargill ordered the plant's temporary shutdown. Perhaps predictably, the company admitted neither fault nor regret. If anything, the later state-ment detailing the new safety measures largely blamed the very workers it failed to keep safe. One *Calgary Herald* colum-nist described the announcement thusly: "It's a doozy filled with whoppers." The company said it had "progressed from encouraging personal face masks to providing them and making their use mandatory"—as if workers had chosen not to engage in health-saving measures. It also said it would work on continued "awareness" of social distancing, inside and out-side work. "This includes," it noted, "not sharing food during meals." Cargill also stressed that it would discourage car-pooling. "We put people first," it added. "No employee should come to work if they are sick or they have been exposed to someone with COVID-19." Even a casual reader did not have to squint to read between the lines: workers' own carelessness and bad (*cultural*) habits, it strongly implied, had caused the outbreak, first and foremost. At the memorial, reporters asked Nguyen if he'd heard from Cargill. No, he said, no condo-lences had come from the company where Hiep had spent more than two decades of her life. A forty-minute car ride away, another worker settled into his wife's spot on the line while Nguyen fought back tears.

Meanwhile, around this same time, in stores across the country, outburst after outburst occurred in the meat aisle. People sputtered over the blank spaces where the ground beef should be. They yelled over chicken breasts and steak cuts and the scared thought of less-than-full bellies. Combined with its other plant in Guelph, Ontario, Cargill has cornered more than 50 per cent of the beef processing market in Canada, and as these and other processing plants shut down, the seemingly endless flow to the shelves trickled. But the situation at Cargill was only the beginning. All over North America, the people who pick Canada's produce and slaughter its meat were not well cared for, their already poor working conditions compounded by a virus that thrives in close quarters and unsanitary conditions. The hard truth is that as some people savoured plump strawberries in sun-beaten parks, barbecued in smoky backyards at six feet apart, and mollified themselves with sugar-crusted pastries, others got sick. These workers fell ill trying to bring you comfort, trying to bring their families comfort, trying to survive.

In April, 184 employees at an industrial bakery in Toronto, which supplies goods to Walmart and Loblaws, got sick. The company, FGF Brands, had encouraged its employees, many of whom are temporary foreign workers, to "get gritty" and make the most of the unprecedented time, during which it boosted hourly pay by a scant fifty cents. "How are you making the most of the disruption?" one company update asked the workers. Like at Cargill, masks were reportedly scarce at FGF in the early days of the pandemic, and social distancing was difficult. But employees kept coming in, even as fear rushed through them, because they couldn't afford not to.

These disease-ripe conditions were repeated at many farms. By early June, more than 420 migrant farm workers had tested positive for COVID-19 across six operations in Ontario. A subsequent report on behalf of over 1,000 migrant workers detailed inadequate food during their mandated quarantine upon arrival to Canada, even worse living conditions (often with one shower to share among upwards of forty workers), and increased surveillance and intimidation. Again, people reported testing positive for COVID but being told to keep working with others who'd also tested positive. As one Jamaican seasonal worker of eleven years said, "We're treated like machines. We just want them to recognize that we're still human."

When she arrived at the Canada–U.S. border, Nicole Folz called Shelley Uvanile-Hesch on a hunch. Uvanile-Hesch is the president and founder of the Women's Trucking Federation of Canada (WTFC), a non-profit that encourages and supports women truckers. She had been off the road since her husband and driving partner, Chris, had died in a workplace accident in August 2019. In the days after taking Folz's call, she would return to the road, driving essential supplies across the country in a fifty-three-foot trailer that, on its sides, featured photos of women frontline medical workers against a hot pink backdrop. It read "STAY HOME SAVE LIVES" and "#FlattenTheCurve." It would be her only drive. As soon as she began the trek, she also began to receive violent threats about the trailer. The wrap also featured the WTFC logo, identifying her. People emailed and messaged on social media to explain, in detail, the harm that would come to her if she crossed into the U.S. They threatened to hurt her wherever they found her. They threatened to run her off the road. She finished the drive in fear and decided she was done. But before any of that happened, Uvanile-Hesch answered her phone. After listening to a distraught Folz, she called Ontario premier Doug Ford on his cellphone. Within ten minutes, Folz had an apology from Public Health Ontario for her ordeal and, at last, a plan.

She pushed her open passport against the window at the crossing and was waved through. Uvanile-Hesch had made sure her load was already cleared to cross. Next, Folz drove her truck back to the yard, sanitized everything, lurched to her car, and drove to a hotel near the Toronto airport that the government had set up for people who, like her, couldn't safely recover at home. She arrived at 9:30 p.m. on Good Friday and felt like she'd walked onto a movie set. Everything was wrapped in white plastic: the walls, ceiling, elevator, floors, tables—all of it. Onsite nurses were dressed in head-to-toe PPE. Folz draped her buffalo plaid shirt over a chair and fell asleep. She was admitted to the hospital the next morning for testing. After one false-negative result, she received her diagnosis: positive. She also received an official letter that informed her she'd have to stay in the hotel for two weeks minimum. When Folz got back from the hospital that day, she decided that other truckers needed to know about her experience. So did younger people who thought the virus would skip over them, like a rock bouncing across water. She pulled up her Facebook profile and began to type: "Wellllll. It happened." She went on to detail her struggle and her symptoms and also posted a photo of her room. In it, a T-shirt-clad teddy bear sat on a white, fleece blanket, emblazoned with the Canadian Red Cross symbol, a loose red thread dangling. Dozens of comments rolled in, hitting over one hundred.

After that brief burst of energy, Folz slept for "three days, pretty much straight." She hardly left her bed, and a nurse visited her three times a day. Medical staff paid particular attention to her temperature, which remained feverish for a week before breaking. At one point, she even got "the whole COVID toe thing." Among the many odd emerging COVID-19 symptoms, including a diminished sense of smell, some people noticed chilblains or frostbite—a condition usually associated with overexposure to cold air. Chilblains are caused by the inflammation of small blood vessels and can cause itching, swelling, blistering, and red or purple patches. In the coming months, there would be considerable medical controversy over "COVID toes," with some studies denying the connection and others supporting it. One study largely surveyed people with no typical symptoms but who suffered from skin lesions. In such cases, the SARS-CoV-2 virus was found in patients' sweat glands and attached to the walls of the skin's blood vessels. Whatever researchers agreed on (or not) didn't matter the night Folz woke up with burning, itching toes, swollen like rows of miniature eggplants. She didn't feel better until the Tuesday of the week after she arrived. She finally ate then, savouring the meal. Soon after, she tested negative.

Folz left the COVID-19 hotel exactly two Fridays after she arrived, at precisely 9:30 p.m. She drove to Bancroft and tiptoed into her house after midnight, home for the first time in months. She knows her dad should have kept his distance, but he heard her—probably wasn't sleeping too soundly, anyway. He bolted out of his bed and hugged her, and pretty soon they were both crying. It was relief, love, something that words can't describe. "My dad is a big softie," said Folz. But even as they embraced, she knew she'd give him something to worry about soon. Folz stayed home for just under a week until she got back in her truck and out on the open road. Her dad, obviously, didn't want her to go. She had a job to do, though, and she tried not to be scared while doing it. People needed supplies and they needed people like her to transport and deliver them. As she drove through Baltimore, through New York, and once again through North Carolina and Louisiana, she was glad to see there were new safety measures and that people kept their distance. She hoped that other truckers were better informed, that their companies and their governments had clear plans in place. She felt alive and excited to be on the road again, freedom zinging through her like Pop Rocks. The feeling of being let down hadn't left her, though, not really, not yet. Without Uvanile-Hesch, and her community of truckers, she didn't know what would have happened.

"THE WEIGHT ON MY SHOULDERS FELT SO ENORMOUS."

Mita Hans,
co-founder of Caremongers-TO

Three

COMMUNITIES COME TOGETHER

Any person entering North Preston, Canada's largest and oldest Black community, will pass a thicket of Maritime wilderness and a burgundy-and-white banner that declares, "We've come this far by faith!" Maybe they'll take a moment to reflect on the community's storied 200-year-plus history, and the people who built it: Black Loyalists who arrived after the American Revolution and slaves who escaped the U.S. during the civil war. Then, they might walk by the long brown-brick elementary school, with the Nova Scotia flag rippling in the grey winds. Or, they'll pass the recently renovated St. Thomas United Baptist Church, maybe pause to listen to the thumping gospel and the hundreds of joyous voices rising up on the air. They might hear a train chugging along the tracks, too, or someone, quite sincerely, telling them they have a beautiful smile. In April 2020, as people travelled further in on the empty streets, however, they likely would have passed something new as well: one of the more than 250 signs reading "During the shutdown of COVID-19, PLEASE NO VISITORS."

The blue-and-red warnings were taped to the front doors of the community's most at-risk homes. "Above all else," they read, "I'm staying home for you. #SpreadLoveNotTheIllness." Thanks to LaMeia Reddick and her fellow advocates, a person walking through the close-knit town that month would also pass another new fixture: North Preston's COVID-19 dedicated testing site—the only place where many of the area's most vulnerable were able to get swabbed for the virus. If they needed to, and many did, they, too, could go in.

Reddick has dedicated most of her adult life to North Preston, the community where she grew up. The twenty-nine-year-old was already in a state of deep grief when a mystery virus began to make headlines. She'd spent the previous months helping care for her sick grandmother, and then, once the cancer completely took over the family matriarch's body, every day mourning her death, fogged in loss. Initially, that's what was real to her, not the virus. She'd taken a break from her advocacy work, at both BLxCKHOUSE, a community centre headquartered in the basement of her family home, and the One North End Community Economic Development Society, a social innovation lab. If you knew Reddick, who is also a community engagement consultant; a founding member of the Change is Brewing Collective, a group lobbying to bring diversity to the food and beverage industry; and often the first to volunteer for a community project, you'd know this sense of stillness signalled just how bottomless her grief was. If you knew her at all, you would also not have been shocked that once she did realize the threat COVID-19 posed to North Preston, she acted.

She laughs when she recalls the moment she realized the potential gravity of the virus. In mid-March, the NBA announced that it would suspend games. She was chatting with one of her family members, who is also a community advocate, who told her the news: "This is real." But little of the public health messaging had reached North Preston—not unusual for the marginalized community, noted Reddick. Indeed, the province's Black communities are notoriously underserviced. Some don't have health care centres. Those that do, such as North Preston, have facilities that often operate on reduced hours. In non-pandemic times these scarce resources can have a disastrous trickle-down effect. For example, one *CMAJ* study showed that, when compared to the rest of the province, the wider Preston area had significantly higher rates of heart disease and stroke, Type 2 diabetes, and mental illness—grim findings that can largely be blamed on poorer access to preventative care and pervasive discrimination within the system. What's more, such disparate findings are not uncommon in Black communities around the Western world. Given that, it's no wonder Reddick, and others in North Preston, had started to ask themselves: how much worse would an already-lopsided system get during a global pandemic?

As she and other community members watched the case counts climb across the country, including in nearby Halifax, following a St. Patrick's Day party, they grew increasingly concerned. They began to think, *Wow, when COVID-19 hits North Preston, it's going to hit hard.* Reddick decided to team up with members of the non-profit ACCE HFX, a collective that supports arts, community, culture, and economics for Black Canadians in the province. Together, they contacted health advocates as well as medical leaders within the Nova Scotia Health Authority and, as a group, formed the Preston Community Response Team. Reddick knew they had to get loud to make sure North Preston would be ready for the virus. Call it a vision, foresight, or a lifetime of experience. She and the others all feared, or maybe just understood, that North Preston and the surrounding communities of East Preston, Cherry Brook, and Lake Loon would be forgotten. Nobody would include them in social distancing awareness campaigns, they wouldn't get good information about community spread or symptoms in a way that spoke to them directly, and the testing sites would be so far away they might as well be on the moon. As one community member would put it, "We don't get much help at all. The little we do have, we have done it ourselves."

Together, Reddick and the other members of the volunteer response team coordinated a push for care. They contacted health authorities to lobby for testing sites. They worked with doctors to learn about the enigmatic virus and its transmission, and then passed on the reliable, fact-based information to everybody they could. They told the system what they needed and how they needed it delivered. On April 7, the

Nova Scotia government finally said it would establish testing clinics in North Preston and East Preston—but the good news did not come without a heavy dose of racism. In his press conference announcing the move, Premier Stephen McNeil followed an age-old pandemic-shaming tactic: he not only blamed the most at-risk and underserved communities for their own poor health outcomes, he suggested they were at fault for everyone else getting sick, too. In breaking previous self-imposed anonymity rules and naming North Preston, he scolded, "And while we are using resources, doubling down on testing, and trying to keep people healthy, the reckless and selfish few in these communities are still having parties. I can't even believe that after everything we've been talking about, some of you think it's okay to have a gathering or a party."

North Preston residents called out the premier's statements for what they were, and he refused to apologize. "We're already fighting the battle of being Black, the battle of being from North Preston," said one resident, Miranda Cain, who had laboured to get the town the resources it needed. "And now we're fighting the battle of being from North Preston and Black and with an infectious disease." That battle didn't slow down after the communities got their testing sites, either. Reddick and the rest of the response team had to work hard to encourage people to get tested. Given the area's harsh history and continued maltreatment, many people understandably distrusted the system now deployed to help them—and the testing site's initial too-small, shabby conditions inside the local

North Preston community centre had only made the hesitancy worse. Reddick joined others in calling friends, family, and acquaintances to assure them it was safe to get tested. She explained the test, what it involved, and why it was so important for people to get it done after others in North Preston had tested positive. Having the response team work with medical professionals, however, did help people get over the hurdle of fear. Reddick said hundreds of residents were tested. It was tough and exhausting, and she was eventually glad when health agencies with more capacity took over the job; she hadn't imagined a full-time job fighting the pandemic. But in that moment she knew it was exactly what she was supposed to be doing. Like hundreds of other women across the country, she'd stepped up to help both her friends and neighbours, as well as people she'd never met, survive. "I kept thinking," she said, "that if we don't mobilize and take the COVID-19 crisis head-on, then we are not going to have a community to do anything for in the future."

The federal government officially launched the Canada Emergency Response Benefit (CERB) on April 6, providing two thousand dollars each month to out-of-work Canadians. The release announcing the program said the cash would help people "put food on the table and keep a roof over their head." To be sure, it was a relief for millions of suddenly jobless Canadians. But the move was also one that had been an agonizingly long time coming. By then, many people had already been without a paycheque for weeks. Others, including the elderly, people with disabilities, those with poor health, and single parents with nobody to watch their kids, couldn't have trekked out to get food even if they did have the funds. All across the country, people struggled toward the possibility of tomorrow. And, incredibly, all across the country others offered what they could. A group of Vancouver activists established a survival fund to dole out no-questions-asked increments of twenty-five to one hundred dollars for things such as electricity bills, groceries, diapers, baby formula. An Indigenous artist named Lianne Spence raised funds to help buy and deliver groceries to elders in the Prince Rupert area. Libraries transformed themselves into foodbanks. And in Toronto, a disability support worker named Mita Hans offered to help one neighbour and unknowingly sprinkled the seeds for a worldwide mutual-aid movement.

Hans grew up in East Africa, or, as she put it, "the area that spawned Ebola." An incoming pandemic means something different, she told me, when your grandfather has had dengue fever—when you yourself remember what childhood malaria felt like. When you know these things in your DNA, then something like a treacherous new coronavirus isn't abstract. It's real. It is "big shit." Hans had been following reports from China. They were vague and disjointed, but all stacked up they felt like something familiar, something dangerous. Hans is also Sikh, and, growing up, when bad things happened her community taught her to ask, "What can I do to help fix this?"

After her family moved to Etobicoke when she was thirteen, Hans organized a fun fair to rally her neighbourhood together. As an adult, following the 2015 terrorist attacks in Paris and a subsequent rise in racism and Islamophobia, she co-created BuddyUpTO. Two men had attacked a Toronto woman wearing a hijab, and the Facebook group allowed anyone who felt unsafe travelling to their destinations to request a buddy. When it comes to helping people, Hans noted, "I've been doing this my whole life." When the pandemic arrived she wasn't about to sit back.

With every new project, Hans asks herself three questions. One: *Who are the most vulnerable?* Two: *What do they need?* And, three: *How can we get it to them?* She started to seriously consider those questions again after knocking on a neighbour's door in mid-March. Hans worried that her neighbour, who has mobility issues and is on the Ontario Disability Support Program (ODSP), wouldn't be able to navigate a packed grocery store or secure the government-recommended two weeks' worth of supplies. Initially, the neighbour tartly told Hans to "stop scaremongering her." Hans replied that she wasn't trying to scare her; she cared. Turning the encounter over in her head later on, near midnight, she began to think about those who would get hit hardest: racialized and Indigenous communities, LGBTQ+ people, the disabled, seniors, the poor and underhoused, everyone on the margins—the same people who always get the knockout blows when crisis comes, compounding already existing issues. She decided to create another Facebook group to connect people who could offer help with the people who needed it. Thinking of the earlier conversation with her neighbour, Hans gave the group a pointedly clever name: Caremongers-TO. She imagined that a couple dozen friends, at most, would sign up to become "caremongers." By March 24, the group had nearly twenty thousand members and was being modelled both across Canada and in thirty-five different countries.

One of those members was Valentina Harper, a fellow activist and friend. Harper grew up in Chile during the dictatorship of Augusto Pinochet and came to Canada during the 1980s. When Hans asked for help with her new project, Harper remembered how, only a month before, Hans had immediately said yes when Harper was grief-worn and needed help— in this case, with emptying her father's house following his death. And so, without thinking too much about it, Harper also said yes. Together, they worked to get advisers from communities that had some of the highest needs. An Indigenous elder signed up, and so did members of the Black Medical Students' Association of Canada. They built a structure that prioritized the most vulnerable and got them the help they needed, without judgment or restrictions. Any person could join the Caremongers-TO Facebook group in their area, post a request, and wait for help to arrive. Many people asked for groceries and other essentials. Others needed face masks, help paying bills or rent, a way to escape an abusive situation, temporary shelter, or medical supplies for chronic conditions.

Later on, some asked for help figuring out their CERB paperwork or talking to their landlord. Anything. Everything.

Day in and day out, Hans and Harper witnessed acts, big and small, that gave them hope. One woman in Mississauga shared that she was down to her last meal for her three children. She hadn't eaten that day at all and she had no money coming in for another week. Hans phoned her and the woman broke down on the call: "I don't know what to do." Hans passed the story on to her sister in Mississauga, who helped the woman connect with their local caremongering group. Within a couple of hours, someone had delivered two Little Caesars pizzas to the woman's front door. Within a couple more, she had $350 in grocery gift cards. People contacted her offering pasta, canned goods, stuff with shelf life. The woman, in turn, contacted Hans again, a new worry on her tongue: "Am I allowed to take it?" Hans told her, "Yes, if somebody offers you something, you take it." That was the whole point. To freely give and receive was something beautiful in the gloom. Hans knows those little moments of generosity helped many donors get through the early months of the pandemic, too. Being isolated at home while others are suffering is a different kind of helplessness; it's an absence of faith, optimism, community, worthwhile tomorrows.

In many ways, it's unsurprising that the idea of caremongering resonated so deeply and so widely. Justin Trudeau tweeted about the movement, saying, "We're only going to get through this by pulling together." Barack Obama called it "a great example of the kind of community spirit we need to get through this." In April, the *Oxford English Dictionary*'s senior editor called *caremongering* her favourite word to emerge from the pandemic, defining the term as: "the provision of help, such as shopping, for vulnerable members of the community during the COVID-19 breakout." She added that it was "a relief to focus on something positive in all the darkness." International media, from the BBC to the *Washington Post*, ran stories about the movement. The former pointed out that Canada is "a country whose inhabitants are stereotyped in the media as being kind to a fault" and called the cumulative #caremongering posts "an uplifting read during anxious times." The latter deemed caremongering "the antithesis in name and spirit to fearmongering." The media storm was intense and often overwhelming, but it wasn't what underscored for Hans how quickly her neighbourhood movement had gone global.

That realization, she said, came when caremongers in Malaysia helped three hundred stranded Rohingya refugees, a group that the UN has dubbed the most "persecuted minority in the world." Though Human Rights Watch has condemned Malaysia's treatment of the thousands who've fled the tyrannical rule in their home country, Myanmar, the caremongers in Malaysia led with defiant kindness. When one member found the refugees in the mountains, too far from any town and begging for water and help, he brought Jeeps full of supplies, donated by other caremongers. In short order, he saved their lives. "And that was the day the magnitude of what we were doing hit me," said Hans. She realized the philosophy of caremongering wasn't only being applied to local challenges, but world-stage tragedies. "The weight on my shoulders felt so enormous. I had a full-on panic attack. I was hyperventilating. This was no longer just a Facebook group. Our actions had very, very real consequences. People's lives depended on how we moved forward." That kind of pressure can make you feel like a bent bough, waiting to crack. Hans and Harper found the increased attention to be heavy and surreal and also, at times, incredibly frustrating.

More than once, they got the chilling sense that both corporate interests and narrowmindedness were co-opting their movement. They saw trendy caremongering T-shirts being sold for profit. And, in some groups, judgment had seeped in like bitter tea. Instead of giving what they could, certain members had started to ask why. To expunge the bad taste, they trademarked the term "caremongering" and began to block and vet members who weren't into giving radical kindness. But it was more than that: too many people were simply missing the point. The problem, wrote Yvonne Su, an assistant professor at York University, is that aw-shucks-Canadians coverage runs the risk of "happy-washing" the pandemic. "While there is an upside to this solidarity, it is often short-lived and romanticized by both media and politicians," wrote Su in an April *Policy Options* piece. "In fact, it may allow the government to download its responsibilities to Canadians and the private sector and abdicate its role in ensuring that everyone is protected and secure." Hans and Harper hadn't started the movement because they were nice Canadians doing nice Canadian things—and they hated to see their movement flattened into a pat-on-the-back moment, especially without discussion of the deeper issues. "The thing is that if Canadians were really nice," said Harper, "we wouldn't be in this predicament."

For many people, the first weeks of the pandemic must have felt like being catapulted into the air, then crashing down, with no safety net in sight. For some, this feeling stretched into months, an endless sense of being Alice in Wonderland, tumbling through infinite strangeness, never once landing. Even worse, they may have looked up as they plunged and seen others cradled in safety: a woven lattice of family, government support, a job, their own savings. It's tempting to blame COVID-19 for this free-falling, but the pandemic only exacerbated inequalities that already existed—snipping the last strings of an already-fraying net. The truth is, a lot of people who felt the worst effects of the pandemic never had much of a net in the first place. Public health messaging around "flattening the curve" urged people to retreat inside. And it worked—but only for the whitest, richest neighbourhoods. For others, it made only slight or no impact. Within the first few months of Canada's national lockdown, what little data there was revealed that in Ontario the rates of infection and death were significantly higher in the province's most ethnically and culturally diverse neighbourhoods. Compared to the least diverse areas, the rate of hospitalization there was four times higher and the rate of death was twice as high. In addition, Toronto discovered that newcomers and those living below the poverty line had higher case and hospitalization rates. Such dismal patterns were echoed in other cities. Contrary to the popular refrain, we were not, it appeared, "all in this together."

The disproportionate statistics make an awful kind of sense. People who live in marginalized and lower-income neighbourhoods often did not have the luxury of working from home. They left their houses every day, risking exposure, because they couldn't afford not to. In particular, racialized women and immigrants made up a lopsided share of those on the front lines, underscoring a long-known wage inequity— they were those who had to keep showing up for work, in large part because they never earned enough money in the first place. When you're making sixty-two cents for every dollar a white man is paid, it's hard, if not impossible, to build an income cushion. Add to that a history of inadequate access to health care, fuelled by a woefully racist medical system, and the reasons behind the disparities become even starker. To afford housing, many lower-income families also live together in smaller dwellings, while others are crammed into crowded apartments and public housing, all places where the virus is at its greediest. And yet, such families still may have fared better than those who were precariously underhoused or homeless during the pandemic. After all, it's also exceedingly difficult to follow the "Stay Home, Save Lives" mantra when you have no home to go to.

Not only was it harder for such people to access hygiene prevention tools, but social distancing meant many shelters were not able to operate anywhere near their usual capacity, even as need increased—in May, one shelter went from handing out three or four hundred meals a week to well over six hundred. It certainly didn't help that people who are homeless tend to have a higher prevalence of chronic health conditions, including heart disease, liver disease, and respiratory issues. Plenty of them are also over sixty-five, the age at which COVID-19 health outcomes become more perilous, more grim. All across the country, many of the services vulnerable populations relied on, including safe consumption sites, day programs, and food banks, were temporarily or permanently shuttered. Fentanyl overdose deaths rose, and many shelters, including those who serve youth, reported being unable to access health care for those who were symptomatic. As the crisis wore on, some cities rented shuttered hotels to help house street-involved populations. In Toronto, a cluster of those hotels were located in the city's higher-income neighbourhoods; protestors rallied to denounce the "criminal element."

Lucy Doan is a nurse practitioner in Toronto. In March, she was midway through a one-year fellowship sponsored by the Medical Psychiatry Alliance. The program is designed to provide better care to people in Ontario who suffer from co-morbid physical and mental health illnesses—two streams of care that are typically, and often disastrously, separated. For the year, Doan rotated through different placements, gleaning all she could about how to give better care. During COVID-19, much of her patient population was racialized, low-income, and living in public housing or relying on the shelter system (or, as the pandemic grew, the expanding tent cities). They may have a diagnosed mental illness such as schizophrenia or may be using antipsychotic medication while also suffering from concurrent chronic illnesses, such as heart disease or asthma. They may also be engaged in substance abuse. In normal times, it's already a vulnerable group that does not usually get the care it needs, she explained. But as spring and silence settled over the city, the situation got even worse. "For the general population, it was like 'Oh my God, it's so awesome that GPs are switching to telemedicine, so care is still accessible and doctors don't have to see you in person,'" said Doan. "But many of our patients don't have homes. They barely have an income—let alone a cellphone or the capacity to access that kind of care. It seemed like the entire population was an afterthought."

She was supposed to stay at her then-current workplace for three months. That tipped into five, putting her on the healthcare front lines of the pandemic everyone seemed to forget. At the start of it all, she matter-of-factly accepted that she would likely contract the virus. She was less worried for herself, though, than she was about becoming an asymptomatic carrier and transporting the virus from place to place like a bad housewarming gift. She knew her clients already had a low baseline of health, and she knew that they'd have a much tougher time accessing care—and worse outcomes—if they did contract COVID-19. The pandemic had destabilized already-shaky ground: some patients battled paranoid delusions, and if they did start exhibiting symptoms, they and many others might also fear going to the hospital. Many such patients also feel stigmatized by the traditional healthcare system. Distrust ran high. Plus, unlike in a hospital, where every patient is treated in a quarantined, vigorously sanitized room and PPE is donned and doffed in crucially sterile settings, the home calls Doan was making required that she dip in and out of poorly maintained and rundown buildings and shelters. She left her own gear on her porch each evening, tied in a garbage bag, and dashed into her house yelling to her husband, "Don't touch me!" She didn't go to the grocery store for months. Risk crackled the air around her.

One day in April (she thinks; everything blended together) Doan changed into her PPE in a creepy downtown alleyway beside a dumpster. A nice, older woman ambled over to chat with Doan and her fellow nurse; they had to frantically ask her to keep two metres' distance. It felt to Doan like she was watching her life from far away, on TV. She made a lot of less-than-ideal wardrobe changes like that, adjusting her armour outside in public spaces before entering high-density buildings. She knew it wasn't proper protocol, but she doused her hands in portable sanitizer and accepted that it was the best she could do. On that particular day, she was making a house call to a woman with a rash. Many of her patients have chronic illnesses that are never addressed and they can be poor historians of their own health, so Doan tries to make as many in-person visits as she can—a seemingly benign symptom can easily be something else. And in this case, it was. Looking at the woman's chart, she realized she had untreated heart failure. After some detective work (a common part of her job), Doan discovered the woman had a GP whom she refused to see. She called the GP and, to her surprise, he also agreed to do a home visit to the woman; he'd been worried about her, too. A few days later, he called Doan to tell her that, when he arrived, the woman's oxygen saturation had dipped to the low eighties. A healthy person is at 92 per cent and above. She was admitted into the ICU and intubated for several weeks. Without intervention, her body would have begun to slowly shut down.

Cases like this haunted Doan throughout the early months of 2020. "What would the outcome have been if I never saw her in person for some rash, never contacted the GP, and he never saw her?" she wondered, even though she already knew the answer. "She would have been dead." She had heard of at least one separate case in which a COVID-positive person who lived in a shelter wasn't intubated at all—if he were someone else, would he have been? She herself had spent one sweltering day, sweating a river through her PPE in an unairconditioned room, trying for nearly two hours to convince a patient to go to the ER. But for every person she caught, how many others slipped through? The helplessness of it all could eat at her. In the public outpouring of gratitude for workers, Doan saw far fewer people delivering free meals and coffee for the nurses and social workers caring for the homeless, thanking them; patients and workers alike were swept under. Doan has never been much of a drinker, and the pandemic didn't turn her into one, but she had also never before finished every shift with a drink, either. She never had more than one drink a day, yet it still felt like a drastic change. She also rented a spin bike and began to exercise constantly. Both distractions numbed her in their own ways.

One Friday spring evening near the end of March 2020, Karen Dougherty was scrolling through social media, thinking about the dire kaleidoscope of images from Wuhan, Italy, New York. As a psychoanalyst and registered psychotherapist, who, at the time, had a practice in Toronto, she worried not only about the virus invading her city but about how the healthcare workers tasked with holding the lines of defence would fare—or, rather, how they were faring right then, watching the virus advance across the globe, unstoppable and untreatable. If SARS-CoV-2 attacked the body, then the pandemic could attack the mind. Depression, anxiety, fear, insomnia, loneliness, stress—each condition could appear in, and even come to define, a healthcare worker's life as the weight of COVID-19 care crushed down. In particular, Dougherty thought about what she and others call "pre-TSD," or, in other words, the anticipation trauma: the worry, "Will it happen here?" and, potentially even more palpitation-inducing, the question, "What will we do if it does?" Talk of a repeat of the SARS outbreak, during which 43 per cent of those who caught the virus in Canada were healthcare workers, was already in the air. So when she saw that a group of New York City mental health practitioners had banded together to offer free mental health services to frontline healthcare workers, her first thought was to fire off a tweet that said, "We should do this here." She barely had time to wonder if people would respond.

Within two and a half hours, someone had helped her make a website and an intake form. Another person helped her put out a call for volunteers. She found her administrator in a friend from grade five whom she hadn't spoken to in forty years. They called themselves the Ontario COVID-19 Mental Health Network. Within two days, 450 licensed therapists had signed on to offer pro bono phone and video sessions to healthcare and social workers in the province. By the end of April, more than 900 registered therapists had signed on to help; Dougherty eventually had to stop taking on new volunteers. They made the process as simple as possible: fill out the form and they'd send you two potential referrals, according to your preferences (maybe, say, you wanted a woman therapist or someone who matched your own racial or cultural background). If you decided not to call, that was up to you. But if you did need to talk to someone, the therapists were there, waiting. Dougherty and her colleagues knew health crises could trigger distress and trauma in healthcare workers, and that the shadow mental health crisis often went untreated. She also felt like the provincial government wasn't ready to step up—in part because "it had no bloody idea this was coming" and in part because it had never rectified the dearth in access post-SARS. She also knew she'd be fighting stigma against accessing mental health care. Whatever the reason, Dougherty didn't want history to carbon-copy itself.

In the end, more than one thousand healthcare and social workers reached out to the grassroots group. Together, their stories were a rushing undercurrent of anxiety, bubbling deep with fear and betrayal, often at odds with the "we got this" narrative the federal and provincial governments presented. Some called to talk about feeling that their hospitals or the provincial government, or both, weren't taking the crisis seriously enough. Many worried that they wouldn't have adequate PPE, or that it would run out, especially those who worked in long-term care homes. Nurses and doctors feared being moved from their regular wards and being made to work exclusively with COVID-19 patients. Their minds chewed on the mystery of it all: Would they know enough to treat patients? What procedures should they follow? How would they keep up with the information, which changed by the day, by the hour? They were terrified of getting sick, and most of all, they were terrified of being the ones who got their families sick. They agonized over the possibility of ventilator shortages and being forced to make gut-wrenching, impossible decisions about who would live and die. And they also worried about regular, everyday human issues that were suddenly, as Dougherty put it, "on steroids." Would somebody's ex-partner use the threat of COVID-19 as an excuse not to let them see their children? Would they not get to say final words to a dying parent? Would lockdown topple a relationship over to divorce?

"That uncertainty is the fabric of anxiety," said Dougherty. "That is what anxiety is." Dougherty is a former full-time documentary filmmaker who began to transition out of the profession after Canadian documentarian Allan King turned to her one day while they were working on a project together and told her she was in the wrong field. Her true calling, he felt, was to become a psychoanalyst. She told him she didn't know what that was, but he persisted. Eventually, she enrolled in a master's program in psychoanalytic studies, while continuing to work in filmmaking, both fields leading her to listen to and document people's trauma, their triumphs, their shaky steps toward healing. After she graduated, she began psychoanalytic training and started her first practice in her Toronto apartment. That was ten years ago. Today, Dougherty makes documentaries about psychoanalysis. She has never lost her belief in the power of storytelling: how it can connect us, unburden our shame, release whatever load we're carrying. She believes at least half the power of it is in the other side— the act of listening to someone's life, of validating that their experiences matter through your own attuned presence.

During the early weeks of COVID-19, she knew she and her

army of listeners couldn't make their temporary patients' anxiety vanish in a few free sessions. Her job, as she saw it, was simply to attend and, in doing so, to help them better tolerate the sense of not knowing, even if only incrementally. That is, after all, what therapists do: they allow people to feel witnessed and heard, to download their anxiety into another person who can contain and detoxify it. Dougherty also hoped that, in some way, she was giving permission for frontline workers to reach out for help, to say that they couldn't handle everything, not always. On the other side of it, her new mental health network gave therapists—many of whom had also had their worlds upended in their own ways—the opportunity to feel like they, too, were using their skills to do something essential. They were healing in their own way. The slow build of everyone recognizing how protecting and cherishing frontline workers' mental health keeps us all alive was worth Dougherty's own long and sometimes stressful days. She couldn't take away the pandemic, but she could let people know they didn't have to endure it alone.

It's tempting to tell the story of women's volunteerism and community engagement during the pandemic as repeated acts of simple selflessness. If, financially, the early days of the pandemic felt to many people like falling without a net, then emotionally, it felt like a giant, sharp-edged spoon, scooping out purpose, scraping down the sides of their lives, shaving away direction, meaning, aim, connection. The social isolation was both abrupt and jarring, cleaving time into *before* and *after*, *normal* and *not*. Some of us stayed home because our privilege afforded it. Millions of others stayed inside because they suddenly had no jobs left to go to. Across the country, we mourned. Across the country, we looked for something to do, something to ward off the sense of feebleness. We wrote hopeful messages in chalk on sidewalks and used kitchen utensils to bang pots and pans at 7 p.m., hoping the colour and the cacophony would communicate connectedness, kindness. We wanted to tell someone everything would be okay; we wanted someone to tell us everything would be okay. It is an incredible quirk of humanity that when things are at their darkest and most chaotic, what gets so many of us through is being able to reach out and help somebody else. Women helped lead so much of that, and while they gained so much, there is always, always a cost.

As the first weeks of the pandemic transformed into the first months, the calls to Dougherty and her team of therapists became less about anxiety and more about burnout. As a therapist, she tries to live by the creed that you have to take care of yourself before you take care of other people. That applies to healthcare workers and it applies to community advocates. Throughout the pandemic, and the uptick in her anxious clients, and the creating and running of an entire help network, Dougherty made sure to create blank spaces in her schedule. She took baths, walked her dog, sewed pandemic quilts, attempted naps. Still, it was easy to leave herself behind, and she recognized that telling frontline workers "take time for yourself" could feel like a ridiculous, terrible panacea. She said it anyway, insisting they figure out a way. And all around the country, her fellow community leaders tried and succeeded, tried and failed to do the same. That's the other way to tell this story of inspiring, life-saving community outreach during the crucial months of COVID-19: that it was hard, and it took a toll. More than that, it exposed how deeply society relies on community advocates to fill gaps. Underneath all that genuine kindness is a type of survival, a sense of being forgotten by the systems that are supposed to take care of you.

Life crushes forward even during a pandemic. Mita Hans's job as a social worker took her on twelve-hour overnight shifts to seniors' community housing buildings. One person whom she cared for contracted the virus just as the caremongering movement catapulted toward fame. During one harrowing night, it didn't look like her client would make it. *This is bad*, Hans remembers thinking, again. *This is not the flu*. Her client survived, but others in her care also got COVID-19. The building had temperature control, but no ventilation, no open windows, no way to leave during a shift. Hans got tested every two weeks, and kept showing up for work every evening, stress hollowing her out, wondering if that would be the night she, too, became sick. Meanwhile, Harper's husband worked on the front line with Toronto's marginalized communities. Harper spent her days volunteering and organizing with Caremongers-TO, looking after their son, working her job as an account manager for a third-party rare book dealer, and wondering if her husband, and everybody else, would be okay. (In fact, the day we all chatted over Zoom, she received a fist-pump-worthy call that he had tested negative.) She had to constantly remind herself that she'd been through worse. Some days it helped and some days it didn't. "We were hurting just like everybody else," Harper said. "We're stressed, just like everybody else. We're anxious, just like everybody else. And we're trying to do this work."

Thousands of kilometres away, LaMeia Reddick was also stressed and trying to do good work. In early March, she was in the process of trying to move out of her mother's house, but good luck finding housing in a newly declared pandemic. She ended up spending a few weeks in a heavily discounted Airbnb in Halifax, telling herself she could use the tough time as a writer's retreat, as a way to recharge. But when she heard there was a shortage of workers for the city's emergency shelters, she signed up for a few overnight shifts as a support worker. As she tried to navigate CERB and reimagine BLxCKHOUSE— obviously, she wouldn't be hosting crowds of people in her mother's house anytime soon—she also tried to figure out the balance between the community's needs and her own. She was still trying to figure it out when a Minneapolis police officer held his knee on George Floyd's neck on May 25, pressing it down and down, even as Floyd said he couldn't breathe, even as it killed him. All the thick, complicated grief she was holding in spilled over, heavy and too much and inescapable. Reddick, characteristically, responded to that dark, tragic moment with community aid, raising twelve thousand dollars to create a fresh, needed pop-up space for BLxCKHOUSE on her mother's driveway and a homework café in the backyard.

There is a word often used to describe people like Reddick: *resilient*. She herself has used the word to describe the community of North Preston. It's in the way the community can lift itself up, can continue to find joy and to love each other and achieve excellence, even through a pandemic, even through endemic racism, even as governments forget and punish and kill them. It's in the way people like Hans, Doan, and Harper reach out to help others, even when they're in danger, even when they want to curl up in a ball and just sleep, or try to. This idea of resilience—of making it through tough times, past obstacles, of bouncing back—is something that Reddick thinks about all the time. She wants to celebrate it, and she wants to conceive where it can take her community once the pandemic is over, what new systems it can create, what hope it might cultivate. There is a lot to learn, Reddick told me, from children who grow up in devastating circumstances and still have bright smiles on their faces. But the other thing about resiliency is that it's complex, she added. It doesn't grow in privilege, in ease, in fairness. "The fact is, why do I have to be so resilient?" asked Reddick. "Why do we not have the basic things that a lot of other communities have?" The fact is, sometimes people have no choice but to go on.

"WE'RE TRYING TO TREAT A DISEASE THAT WE BARELY KNOW ABOUT."

Dr. Kanna Vela,
emergency room physician

Four

VIRUS ON THE FRONT LINE

Before the first patient arrived in New York or Madrid or Toronto, Janet Pilgrim believed the new coronavirus outbreak would be like the first one. When SARS hit Canada in 2003, Pilgrim was a frontline nurse at Toronto Western Hospital's emergency department. She remembered the fear and isolation and the sense that death was riding in. At the time, she was set to get her driver's licence in nearby Mississauga, but after learning she was a nurse in the city, her instructor refused to teach her. Friends wouldn't let her enter their houses. Forget frontline hero; she became a pariah. It was like her breath was a loaded weapon, every exhale a grenade. Nearly everybody was afraid she would expose them to the virus and that they, in turn, would spread it to their families. She was afraid for her family, too. Her children were only two and three years old, a particularly vulnerable age for SARS. Her colleagues were getting sick. Some were dying. The so-called killer bug had largely caught the healthcare system off guard, and everyone knew it. The news channels blinked panic, people in masks on the street, comatose patients on stretchers.

In early 2020, those memories piled into pyramids and, thinking back, Pilgrim thought she had an understanding of what was coming. She also thought the hospital was well-prepared to handle it. She had now been at the hospital for three decades, and had advanced to nurse manager of general internal medicine ward 8B. Her team of sixty had successfully managed various outbreaks at the downtown hospital over those years, including H1N1 in 2009. Controlling the new virus wouldn't be easy, but her team worked well together, was highly skilled, and had done it before—or so they thought. Along with leaders at the other hospitals within the University Health Network (UHN), the umbrella under which Toronto Western and several of the city's other sites sit, Pilgrim began strategic planning and collaborated on emergency preparedness guidelines and protocols. As news blighted Wuhan, hospital leaders decided they needed a uniform response. This time, there would be neither pockets of failure nor pockets of excellence. Every precaution and procedure would be unveiled at the same time, on the same day, in the same way. People from across all departments of all the hospitals collaborated, planning meticulously, examining every angle, determined not to jeopardize frontline healthcare workers again. Pilgrim remembers assessing the plans and thinking, *We've done a good job.* That confidence was fleeting.

"By the time the virus truly came through the doors of Canada," said Pilgrim, "the world was in a pandemic." SARS had caused havoc on two continents. In contrast, the emerging coronavirus had eclipsed the globe. *Oh. My. Goodness,* thought Pilgrim, each syllable an anvil thudding sand. *How has it already impacted so many?* Almost overnight, people became consumed with counting COVID-positive cases, with counting deaths. Hospitals in Europe were running out of beds in their intensive care units (ICUs). PPE was in dangerously low supply, seemingly everywhere. A shortage of ventilators meant doctors had to decide who would live and die, their days bloated with impossible choices. Pilgrim watched the accelerated advance and realized this new virus wasn't like SARS at all. That virus was unquestionably deadly and awful, but it was also fathomable—it happened on a scale the human brain could understand. *This* virus was what people called it: a wave. One so big it felt biblical, threatening to scrub the world clean. Whatever careful plans the hospitals had made, she now knew they needed to work on additional plans. Maybe they were barely prepared at all. And every second they failed to fix that could add a blunt tick to the world's new death-watch obsession.

In response to this realization, a physician within the UHN reached out to a doctor in Spain who was tweeting about his hospital's COVID-only units. By then, the European country had outpaced mainland China's death toll, coming second only to Italy. Healthcare workers in Canada had no reason to believe they wouldn't suffer the same dismal fate if they didn't learn from the mistakes made in the rest of the world. Doctors in Madrid gladly shared the harsh lessons they'd learned, those in turn imbued with grim knowledge from Wuhan. Soon, Pilgrim and her colleagues had a new plan. They decided to reorder the hospital into taped-off, colour-coordinated risk zones, reminiscent of a basketball court. Staff drew red lines around individual patient rooms, indicating extremely high contamination danger. Nurses and doctors inside the red zone must wear PPE and must also take it off before exiting. The intermediate-risk green zone was where everyone put on their hygiene armour. The nursing station itself sat in the blue, or "super clean" zone, which nobody could enter without washing their hands. They drafted safety checklists, practised patient visits, learned how to work PPE with nursing partners, drafted post-round checklists. Over and over again, they rehearsed for disaster.

"And then reality hit," said Pilgrim. On a Friday afternoon—because bad news is always delivered on a Friday, something Pilgrim vowed right then to change—her clinical director told her that her ward would be the designated COVID-positive unit. The words knocked around in her suddenly hollowed-out chest, again: *Oh. My. Goodness.* She had spent the preceding weeks psychologically preparing for the pandemic. But it's one thing to steel yourself, and quite another to tell your team they're going to war. Fear throttled the entire world, and at the time, Toronto Western was no different. She gathered the afternoon shift inside a room. As a nurse and a team leader, Pilgrim has had to deliver some pretty tough information. This was the hardest. She wasn't just saying, *Prepare for a rough few weeks at work*. Read between the lines and the message was, *Prepare for death*. "Okay guys," she told the assembled crew. "I have some news." Pilgrim tried a positive spin: because of their stellar work on previous flu outbreaks, and their famil- iarity with PPE, hospital administration had designated them as the COVID ward. When she finished, the room went silent. She could see the fear etched on their faces. Tears slipped.

They were afraid for their families. What if they passed it on to their elderly parents? What if they took it home to their husband, their child? How would they keep *everybody* safe? The questions collapsed into each other, and Pilgrim sifted through the rubble of fear, rescuing each concern, addressing every fear. Inside, she felt their pain. On the outside, she made a mantra of reassurance: we know how to do this, we are a strong team, we can make it through together; we are nurses, we are professionals, we will offer professional care. "Let's pause," she said. "Let's remember what we know." Eventually, she felt everybody begin to breathe again. After they left, Pilgrim stayed behind and had the same wrenching conver- sation with her night staff. When dawn crested, she told her morning staff—a déjà vu of clawing fear, panic, resolve.

As Pilgrim prepared her ward, about an hour's drive away, in Hamilton, Cathy Risdon sat down to write three emails. Risdon is a vice-chair in the Department of Family Medicine at McMaster University, and the school's director of health services. She's been in the department itself for over twenty years, focusing on building collaboration, communication, and professionalism within the medical field. She'd need all those skills now as she tried to distill one of the most catastrophic, unprecedented crises in modern history. Even as most of us were compassionately, robotically swapping "Cheers" and "Best" for "Stay safe" and "Be well," to Risdon the once-simple act of emailing felt loaded, impossible. What do you say when safety and wellness are so deeply uncertain, so compromised— especially for those on the front line? Risdon's first email to her physicians and residents was, more or less, the warm-up act. She explained the importance of handwashing and talked about the power of prudent care in protecting the community. The second email, sent about ten days later, praised their work. She told her staff they were doing a great job and commended the way they were mobilizing and looking out for each other.

But as she sat down to write her third email, the world felt like a different place. *There are people in our professional circles, and in our clinics, that could die from this*, she thought. The slimmest of margins, and a whole lot of luck, might be the only thing stopping Hamilton or Toronto or Vancouver from becoming New York or all of Italy. It was the lull before SARS-CoV-2 had infested Canada. People might have wanted to use the pause to grow sourdough starters, or learn a new language, but what they really should be thinking about, she became convinced, was if their wills were up to date. Risdon began to type: "Based on the experiences of other countries, we need to be prepared for the possibility that some very hard, sad things will happen to people in our work circles and our family circles." Warning of overwhelmed hospitals and a shortage in care, she continued: "A lot may happen without our ability to prevent or control it." The best thing her staff could do now was break the taboo on discussing death—before it was too late. "Do you have a will?" she asked her staff, encouraging them to have an honest, compassionate conversation with their loved ones. "Powers of attorney for finance and personal care? Are all your insurance policies and financial documents organized and easy to find?" If the worst happened, what kind of death did they want?

She pressed send. "I'm not one for candy-coating everything," she told me. "And, it certainly provoked strong reactions in all directions." Some of her staff felt grateful that she had broached the subject in such a direct, open manner. Others wished they'd been given a warning that they, and their own staff, were about to have a frank conversation about what might be ahead. Knowing would have allowed them to better support the staff that was already freaked out, they told Risdon. She thanked them for their feedback—it was a fair point. But she doesn't regret sending the email; she needed to acknowledge the gravity of the situation. And it was grave. Throughout March and April, Risdon's days felt soaked in terror. Months later, when I speak to her during the summer of 2020 as Canada's daily case counts dipped, she almost laughs at that word, *terror*. Removed from those early weeks, it feels like such a dramatic choice. But she also can't deny that's what it was. She worried that the healthcare system in Canada might make the same mistakes as elsewhere: namely, sending every sick person to the hospital, neglecting both primary and at-home care, and creating accidental hotspots. She worried that both COVID tents and testing centres would enable the virus to cluster and spread. One wrong step could wreck every good, careful intention. She worried that hospitals, public health agencies, and other medical experts wouldn't get it right.

"I feared that our actions would make us have a COVID tsunami," Risdon said. "It was this actual terror that we would be the inadvertent authors of our own demise."

In the early months of the pandemic, Cora Mojica learned a lot about feeling terror. Mojica immigrated to Canada from the Philippines in 1987, leaving behind both her training as a secretary and most of her extended family. For the first two years, she was employed as a nanny. After she was granted permanent residency, she moved over to shipping and receiving, working at the same company for thirteen years before being laid off. In 2004, she applied for a job at the company that staffs hospitality workers at Vancouver General Hospital. Mojica got the job and has been there ever since. Her hospital is the city's biggest, and on any given day she and her co-workers may have to prepare specialized meals for over one thousand patients. They're not a team of superwomen, and sometimes they have to talk to their supervisor about whether they can make all those meals, fill all those trays. But, on a good shift, there's a certain kind of regularity to the job—a coordinated dance to the clinking of cutlery, the fast-paced knock-clunk of dishes. Each day, there are about sixty food staff working, including cooks, bakers, and those prepping and placing food in the tray line. For each meal, Mojica's team has two tray lines running at the same time, with ten people working each one. Some people fill the tray and the others move the food around the hospital, chugging metal wagons. Mojica is responsible for placing the milk and juice. Another person ladles the soup, snatches the crackers, chooses the dessert. One grabs the right pieces of each entrée. A symphony of breakfast, lunch, and dinner.

When we think of healthcare workers, we often imagine physicians, nurses, technicians, specialists, surgeons—people who've dedicated their lives to helping the sick, the injured, and the dying. We think of clipboards and scalpels, scrubs and prestige. For the vast hospital enterprise to work, however, it also needs an army of cleaners and sanitizers, people to feed all those patients trying to get better, security guards to make people feel safe. In the uncomfortable hierarchy of health care, these key workers are often near the forgotten bottom and they are often, uncoincidentally, members of vulnerable populations. Many of them make not much more than minimum wage. Mojica estimates that 90 per cent of her co-workers are women of colour, and that the vast majority are from the Philippines, like her. In fact, across the system, immigrants play a vital role in Canadian health care, accounting for one out of four workers. A virus doesn't have feelings; it doesn't make a distinction between the person who intubates a rapidly declining patient and the person who wipes down their room after that last-ditch effort fails. Its one goal is to invade, replicate, take over. In those early months, every single person who walked into a hospital was also trekking into the virus's hostile breeding grounds. All of them could get sick. And disproportionately, they did.

By mid-May, in Ontario, healthcare workers comprised 17 per cent of all COVID-19 cases in the province, up from 10 per cent the month before. The vast majority of them were workers like Mojica: non-medical staff who showed up every day for their shifts, many of them because they couldn't afford not to. (The first healthcare worker who died in the province was a hospital cleaner.) Mojica herself told me, more than once, that as scared as she was—as scared as she knew everyone on her shift was—she was also grateful to still have a job during the pandemic. This gratitude kept her going through the fear; not having an income was worse. "Even though it's hard," she said, "we still have to be grateful we have a job because others don't." Even those on CERB, she added, could be suffering more than those on the precarious front lines. "They have a family, they have a mortgage, they have to put food on the table," she added. "Just do the job," she told herself and her worried colleagues, not unkindly. "Just do the job."

Elsewhere in the world, a *Lancet* study published in late July confirmed that healthcare workers in the U.S. and the U.K. were at a far higher risk of contracting the virus than the generalized population. More alarmingly, it also showed that Black, Asian, and other people of colour in the healthcare field were at an even higher risk—five times more so than the (white) generalized population. A joint Guardian and Kaiser Health News project, Lost on the Frontline, identifies healthcare workers who died from COVID-19. In August, it estimated 62 per cent of the healthcare workers it catalogued were people of colour. The cause of the jaw-dropping disparity, the *Lancet* authors found, is multi-pronged failure. Many racialized healthcare workers were more likely to work in settings with greater exposure to patients with COVID-19, whether it be a designated ward, a busier hospital, or a long-term care centre. They were also more likely to receive inadequate PPE, or none at all, or to be asked to reuse what they did have. More research into the inequality, added the authors, was "urgently needed."

Mojica didn't need a study to know the risks. She felt them in her own fluttering fear, saw them etched in the faces of her scared colleagues. It wasn't only the hospital setting itself that could seem like a losing gamble. Mojica doesn't have a car and so rides the bus every morning for her 10:30 shift. Before Vancouver declared a state of emergency, it would take her about an hour to get to work. During the lockdown, it took at least two hours. Sometimes, she'd watch one, two, three crowded buses go by before it was safe enough for her to board. Other times, she'd have to call a taxi. The worst was when she found a seat on the bus only to face racist vitriol. Twice, with her mask on Mojica was mistaken for a Chinese woman. One Canadian poll, released in June by Angus Reid and the University of Alberta, showed that half of those within Asian communities had experienced racial slurs or insults because of the pandemic's geographic origin. Another 43 per cent said they had faced threats or intimidation. Racist graffiti blared from tunnels and underpasses, boarded-up shops, street signs. It filled our social media feeds and escaped the mouths of world leaders. Strangers blamed Mojica for bringing the virus to the city; they told her to go back home. Normally, she's an outspoken person, but this time she bit her tongue, asking the Lord to forgive the racists. "Even though I'm not Chinese, it hurts," she said. "Because why, why, *why* would anyone say that to people?"

At work, her manager updated the team on the increasing COVID-19 case counts before every shift. Workers who were dropping off food had to wear full PPE. In COVID-19 wards, they were no longer allowed to enter the patients' rooms. Once they arrived outside the ward that separated them from hopeful safety and definite danger, they had to phone a nurse who would don their own PPE and enter the room. The tray, plates, cups, and cutlery were all now paper or plastic, completely disposable. But the food cart would have to go back down, sanitized once before it travelled through the corridors and on the elevators, and then again when it arrived back in the kitchens. During her breaks, she ate alone, following the new protocol. Even with all the extra cleaning and precautions, even with all her gratitude, Mojica still felt afraid sometimes. Her routine became work–home, work–home, work–groceries–home, repeat. Mojica is a widow and lives by herself, and during those wiped-out nights at home she would often FaceTime her mother and siblings in the Philippines, who were fifteen hours ahead. She'd tell them to wear a mask, not to socialize, and to keep the required six feet of distance. It was impossible to tell who could be a carrier, she told them. You could be walking around with no symptoms, never even knowing you were orchestrating death. She worried about them, constantly.

One of the most frightening things about SARS-CoV-2 is its often puzzling stealth. The virus's predecessor is more like a blustery relative, loudly announcing itself—a characteristic that, in many ways, provided the strategy for its defeat. SARS-CoV was, and remains, deadly and highly contagious, traits it shares with the virus that causes COVID-19. Unlike its fellow coronavirus, however, SARS-CoV by and large makes people obviously very sick. It's also only contagious when a person has symptoms. The virus weasels its way into a victim's lungs and triggers horrible coughing, thus rowdily launching itself out of said person's mucus-ways and onto the next victim. The resulting droplets are relatively heavy and do not travel far. During the height of the SARS outbreak, all of this made it easy to identify when a person was infectious and, in turn, easy to isolate them, then contact potential next victims and isolate them too. Little of that is true for SARS-CoV-2. During the first wave, it was still unclear how easily pre-symptomatic and asymptomatic people could transmit the virus. It was also unclear just how many of those people existed. But what was clear was that they *did* exist. As some people died startling, sudden deaths after becoming infected with SARS-CoV-2, others went on living, feeling no different at all.

After half a year of research, scientists were still recording wildly different answers on the prevalence of asymptomatic cases. The WHO reported that the share of true asymptomatic cases ranged anywhere from 6 to 41 per cent. The huge variance can partly be blamed on another difference in the virus's transmission and presentation: pre-symptomatic carriers who display no symptoms but who will go on to. This population can also spread the virus, walking around for days and feeling fine as it invades their body and sends out minuscule scouts. The U.S. Centers for Disease Control and Prevention (CDC) has estimated that 40 per cent of SARS-CoV-2 transmission has happened before people even feel ill. In other words, when it comes to the virus, the traditional wisdom about disease spread and control no longer applies. It has seemed to evade patterns just as easily as it does detection. It lodges high levels of particles in the nose and mouth, making it particularly easy for the replicating viral soldiers to escape into the environment—a process called viral shedding. The simplest way for the virus to do this is when a person coughs or sneezes, but studies have also shown the virus can shed when a person talks, shouts, or sings. What's less certain is how long the virus can survive suspended in air or on surfaces (creating what's called a fomite). When it comes to the latter, research during the first wave showed the virus can survive for hours or days, depending on both the environment and the material of the surface or object.

"There are so many unknowns," confessed Maria Van Kerkhove, the WHO's technical lead for coronavirus response and head of its emerging diseases and zoonoses unit, in June. And in the absence of a scientific answer on where the virus skulked, or just how dangerous it could be to find it, another answer emerged: clean everything. By spring 2020, we were all experts in handwashing, dutifully singing the entirety of "Happy Birthday" as we scrubbed between our raw, cracked fingers. We plowed through Lysol wipes and sloshed bleach on everything. We zealously washed our groceries, the bottoms of our shoes, our jackets, takeout containers, plastic bags, our dogs. News stories emerged of third-party sellers charging $184.99 for bottles of hand sanitizer on Amazon.ca and $40 for bottles of travel-sized Purell on eBay. Even brick-and-mortar stores upped their prices to cover costs after shortages forced them to seek out new, more expensive suppliers. The astronomical inflation didn't stop shoppers from stocking up; whole shelves went empty as people became desperate to acquire what scant protection they could. In hospital settings, where sick patients were already vulnerable to infection, janitorial and housekeeping work took on new weight. Doctors and nurses could follow distancing protocol and blue-green-red lines on the floor, but the deeper, daily work of keeping everyone safe fell to lower-paid cleaners.

Precy Miguel has been employed as a housekeeper at St. Paul's Hospital in Vancouver since 2006. By 2020, she'd been working in the emergency department for two years. When COVID-19 patients arrived at her hospital, she was scared, just like everybody else. She'd see patients intubated in their rooms and know that, at some point, she'd have to enter that same room to clean it. She tried to fill her heart with positivity and optimism. *We can fight this*, she'd tell herself, donning her N95 mask, face shield, goggles, and gown. *We can do it.* She was skilled and she had the gear and there was no way she could get infected if she followed proper protocols. She willed herself to believe it every time she read a sign on a patient's door telling her how sick they were, how high her risk was, what she had to put on before heading in, everything she had to spray and wipe and mop. All around the world, people were dying and if she really loved her neighbours—and she did— then she had to clean the rooms where the virus waited. "We have to clean," she told me. "We have to sanitize so that we can get rid of this crisis." The thought of saving just one person kept her going through the fear.

In March and April, both extra duties and staffing shortages meant Miguel would often have to work a double shift—her seven and a quarter hours stretching to nearly fifteen. Some-times, she worked every day of the week, reminding herself that she was doing what needed to be done. Certain days were tougher than others. Miguel lives with her elderly parents and two brothers, and has been sleeping in the living room during the pandemic, behind a partition, to add extra distance. Her mother is unwell and during the pandemic was admitted to Miguel's hospital for more than a week, luckily not with COVID-19. Nurses let Miguel visit once, but she mostly stuck to phoning her mom, following the hospital's safety measures. Her mother worried that nobody visited her, wondered why she was alone in her hospital room, cut off from the comfort of family. Miguel tried to explain that it was for her own good, but was relieved when her mother was released. She remained meticulous about her cleaning routine. After every shift, she put her uniform in a plastic bag and changed into fresh scrubs. Once through the doors of her building, she sanitized every-thing in her path, as well as herself. Sometimes, after working a double shift, she'd be too exhausted to begin her next cleaning ritual and would spend the night sleeping in her car. She'd seen the patients in the COVID-19 rooms and didn't want any-body in her family to end up like that, silent and unconscious as she killed the virus around them.

Miguel is also the chair of her union local, and spent much of her time in that role adopting a brave face and fielding others' concerns. Between focusing on her work duties, her family, and her co-workers, she barely had time to think about how she herself was faring during the pandemic. Her brothers are also essential workers, and Miguel insisted on not deviating from her usual grocery-shopping routine for the family. She also takes care of the building in which they live, and spent hours cleaning the railings, doorknobs, everything— you might as well add the tenants to her list of responsibilities. Her mind circled around those she cared for and about, looping the questions, *What else can I do for them? What more is there? How can I still help?* Often, she'd add another lap to her concerns by worrying about her family back home in the Philippines. The more scraped thin her energy became, the more she reminded herself: *If nobody will clean the hospital, how can we save those people?* Yes, she needed her paycheque, but that wasn't why she stayed. She stayed because she knew she had an important role to play in controlling the pandemic. It was her job to stop it from getting anyone else sick. Once it was in the body, well, then it was already beyond her control.

First, the nanny quit. Dr. Kanna Vela had hired her to look after her young children, ages five and two and a half, while she worked the emergency departments at three different hospitals in the Greater Toronto Area (GTA). She used to run a busy family practice, too, for seven years, back before her second daughter was born. She loved it, but she quickly realized it left her with little time to see her children and made the difficult decision to move full-time to emergency medicine. Even her most chaotic shifts were regimented in strict slots during the evening, night, and early morning, leaving her precious hours with her kids while they were both still awake. Vela and her husband, who runs a software company, were making it work—until March and the pandemic and their nanny's understandable need to be at home with her own children. Vela wasn't sure it was even safe for her to be in her own house. She'd surely be working with COVID-19 patients, and the last thing she wanted was for her family to become some of them. So, along with her parents, she devised an elegant, heart-breaking solution: she'd move into their home, and they'd move into hers. Her daughters would be cared for and Vela would be alone.

For weeks, she didn't see her family at all. Her husband read the girls their bedtime stories and tucked them in, while Vela read medical journals and attended hospital Zoom meetings. Eventually, it became unbearable. Though she knew there wasn't much science to back up her decision—there still wasn't very much science on the virus at all—she started making trips home on the third day of her three-day weekly break, so long as she felt well for the first two. There, she'd be sure to socially distance from her parents, playing a sort of musical chairs through the house, from the kitchen to the family room to the living room. Back at her makeshift home, she followed an elaborate sanitization routine—one she stuck with when, two months later, she finally moved back in with her family.

Like many frontline staff treating COVID-19 patients, she avoided eating or even drinking water through most of her shift because the risk of removing her mask at the hospital was too high. At the end of her shift, she'd change at the hospital, then strip out of the clothes she wore home from work in the garage, and either tie them up or put them in the laundry right away. Then she'd run naked up to the shower. Nobody else could use her bathroom, just in case the steam from the hot water was infected and helped the virus aerosolize. Afterward, she'd use a Lysol wipe to clean anything she might have touched: her keys, her phone, doorknob handles. It took at least forty-five minutes, added on to the lengthy decontamination procedure she already did at the hospital. Sometimes, she wouldn't make it home until 3 or 4 a.m., barely able to drag her body to the shower. "You can easily forget things when you're tired and stressed," she said. "And then you spend the next day worrying, like, 'Did I miss a step? Will that mean someone at home gets sick?'"

To help cope with the uncertainty, Vela focused on what she could control. Every healthcare worker in Canada had the perverse advantage of watching the pandemic unfold elsewhere first—the virus might have been sketched in question marks, but Canadian workers had more information than those in other countries did when they started. And they knew, if they were to have any chance, they needed PPE. Instead of waiting to run out of N95 masks, Vela and a few colleagues started a PPE drive. She got her husband to make a website. Another doctor reached out to CP24, the local news station, to talk about the drive. They urged chiropractors, dentists, family doctors, and any other medical office that was closed to donate their masks. "Yours will come," they urged them, "but we need them right now." Medical students volunteered to do inventory, and another doctor offered up their empty clinic to store the bounty. Word of mouth spread and people crafted face shields; Vela and her colleagues scoured the city for extra stock, for protection normally used in other, industrial fields. Fear threaded through those moments. Vela refused to let it paralyze her; action became an antidote.

It all helped, but it didn't cure the frustration and the trauma of not quite knowing how to treat her patients. "We're trying to treat a disease that we barely know about," Vela said—a disease, she added, that had no treatment. "That can be very hopeless." Too much of her job was reduced to guesswork and supportive care. The constant surprise of helplessness gnawed at her. So too did watching patient after patient die alone, with nobody to hug them, to hold their hand, or to place a gentle, final kiss on their brow. That was true of all end-of-life patients during those months, whether they had COVID-19 or not. Sometimes a loved one could say goodbye through a tiny window slit. Later on, they could FaceTime through a donated iPad. Vela knew it wasn't enough. And she ached to know she couldn't give them, or their families, the dignified, full deaths they deserved. Sometimes she'd think about the already-emerging group of pandemic deniers and think about whether they'd still believe it was all a hoax if they could shadow her through the hospital, see the same sickness and grief that she did. If they could feel what it was like to try everything to save someone and still have it feel like throwing dice in Vegas.

By April, the only thing that seemed certain about SARS-CoV-2 was that it did not act like any other coronavirus. "It can attack almost anything in the body with devastating consequences," said one U.S.-based doctor that month. "Its ferocity is breathtaking and humbling." A subsequent research paper published in the *Lancet* termed the stages of infection as "the four horsemen of a viral apocalypse." It deemed the first horseman a "sneaky virus." That virus, doctors and scientists knew, entered through the lining of the nose, where it found a lush expanse of cells that have a cell-surface receptor called angiotensin-converting enzyme 2, or ACE2, which is usually responsible for regulating blood pressure in the body. It also marks tissue potentially vulnerable to infection, and SARS-CoV-2 needs it to enter a cell. (In fact, any virus that infects animals needs the right cell receptor to infect—think of them as carrying, or perhaps stealing, the right key for the corresponding receptor lock.) After that, the virus begins its endless chain of reproduction and invasion. This can cause the more well-known symptoms of COVID-19: dry cough, sore throat, achy body, loss of smell and taste, fever. In the Bible, the first horseman is the Antichrist, riding in on a white horse, sowing disruption and readying the world for the other three—war, famine, death. If the body's immune system doesn't beat back the first horseman, things get similarly grim.

The virus will continue down the weakened body, travelling the windpipe to attack the lungs. The lung's so-called respiratory tree ends in tiny air sacs called alveoli. A single layer of cells rich in ACE2 receptors lines each one—an irresistible home for the virus to ransack. This is when SARS-CoV-2 can turn deadly. As the immune system tries to defeat the virus, the resulting battle inhibits the healthy, normal flow of oxygen. Then come the classic pneumonia-like symptoms: pitching fever, coughing, a struggle to breathe. Sometimes, with medical intervention, such as a ventilator or even oxygen through simple nasal prongs, a patient can get better. Other times, most times, the battle between immune system and virus pushes a body toward rapid, baffling deterioration. An estimated 80 per cent of those infected with the virus remain asymptomatic, or only develop minor or moderate illness. They stay home, they isolate, and they get better. The other 20 per cent get sick enough to require hospital admission. And 5 per cent of those end up on ventilators, silently, unconsciously fighting for their lives in the ICU.

In the first months of the pandemic, there seemed to be no way to tell which path a body would follow, or how to intercept the last horseman in any analogy: death. Compounding the unpredictability—the maddening senselessness of it all— was the virus's tendency to sometimes travel, and invade, any part of the body with ACE2 receptors. Usually, the chief mandate of a coronavirus is to reach the lungs. But SARS-CoV-2 can also target the kidneys, which have ample ACE2 receptors, and which, if infected, significantly heighten the risk of death. Sometimes it kept travelling down, to the intestines, causing diarrhea. Other times it targeted the liver, messing with enzyme levels. Some of the sickest patients developed pink eye. More rarely, the virus will make its way to the brain, which houses ACE2 receptors at its neural cortex and stem. It can invade them, but it can also suffocate nearby cells, sucking up needed oxygen and causing them to die. Neurological invasion can cause strokes, seizures, confusion, headaches, and delirium. At its deadliest, the virus seems insatiable, overtaking every part of the body it can. Some studies have suggested that pre-existing conditions, like asthma and diabetes, the size of the initial viral load, and age may provide clues as to how sick a person will get. Even with those scientific hints, however, concrete answers remained evasive.

"We see these weird cases, and we can't just say, 'Oh, it's just elderly who are at high risk' or 'it's just patients who have other medical conditions,'" said Vela. "It would be easier if this disease followed rules." Every doctor or nurse who treated COVID-19 patients seemed to have at least one case they couldn't make sense of. For Vela, it was a man with a young family, who had returned from travel in March, and, as far as they could tell, had no major medical problems. He had come to the COVID-19 clinic after his cough and fever worsened. Staff at the clinic thought he didn't "look so good" and sent him to Vela's emergency department. She swabbed the man for the virus, did some blood work, and took some X-rays.

It seemed likely he had the virus, but his vitals were stable and his X-rays looked okay. She sent him home to isolate, but also took his name and number so she could call him immediately with his results. There was no scientific reason for her worry— she just had a bad feeling. When his test came back positive the next day, she called him. He was still coughing, but he wasn't short of breath, the tell-tale sign of a worsening case. They decided he could stay at home and keep resting. But Vela couldn't shake her apprehension. She called him the next day, and the day after that. On the fourth call, she noticed a difference in his speech pattern, a shortness of breath. She told him to come back, paused, and said, "Actually, call 9-1-1." He needed an ambulance. She warned him that she'd call back to make sure he had; she didn't want to hear about any stereotypical male stubbornness.

As soon as he arrived at the hospital, he was put on oxygen. His X-rays were covered with white splotches; black areas represent air. Shortly after, doctors intubated him and put him in the ICU, where he only got worse. Within a few days, they transferred him to Toronto General Hospital, which has an extra-corporeal membrane oxygenation (ECMO) machine. Considered to be the next level of therapy for COVID-19 when everything, even a ventilator, has failed, an ECMO machine is the most aggressive form of life support available. It pumps and oxygenates blood outside the body, then returns it—in this case, doing the work of the lungs when a patient's own have stopped working. It can perform miracles, but it just as often doesn't work. Vela followed the man's case from afar; he had small children at home and, painted in the broadest strokes, he reminded her of her husband, or even herself. He was relatively young, generally healthy, and they'd gone over and above with his care, calling him at home, pushing him to come in. Surely, if anybody could make it . . . The thought hurt too much to finish. But he didn't make it. When Vela found out he had died, she did the only thing she could now do: she cried.

And sometimes, just as puzzlingly, a patient survived. During the first wave, Janet Pilgrim's COVID-19 ward at Toronto Western Hospital became a busy place, ebbing between hope and devastation. Most of her twelve-hour days were emotionally draining. She still ran every meeting with her ward's three shifts. She continued to comfort nurses, even as they moved into a slow, steady routine—carefully, deliberately donning PPE before entering any patient's room. Together, they figured out how to care for patients who all had the same disease but not always the same symptoms. Together, they watched people die.

And together in October 2020, they also weathered an outbreak in the hospital that would temporarily close Pilgrim's ward. It was the hospital's sixth and, at that point, worst outbreak; by the end of October, the cumulative outbreaks had infected thirty-eight patients and sixty-eight staff. Pilgrim later said of the intense time, "I went on autopilot—there was no time to feel upset or distraught." She had work to do: moving patients out of the ward, ensuring a "terminal clean," directing her staff, trying to keep everyone safe.

The stress, the fear, the long days were all worth it, though, when someone reversed the expected story and walked out of the hospital. The first patient to deteriorate quickly in Pilgrim's ward was a seventy-six-year-old man who, she recalls, was quite sassy. He was transferred to the ICU, where he stayed on a ventilator for a month. After he was transferred, so were five other patients, in short, bleak succession. She didn't think he would return, but he did—delighting the staff with freewheeling stories of his life as they helped to rehabilitate him. When it was time for him to be discharged, she gathered all the nurses on her ward, the physicians, the clinical director, everyone. As he walked out, they formed a wall of support, clapping so hard and for so long their hands probably turned red. He clapped, too. Pilgrim remembers looking around and seeing people crying. But this time they were elated. They clapped out the next patient and the next and the next. They did it for the patient and they did it for themselves, a reminder that they weren't so helpless after all.

As a nation, we have widely celebrated healthcare workers as heroes, particularly during the initial months of the lockdown. Corporations offered stacks of online discounts, stores offered front-of-the-line privilege, restaurants donated scores of food. Those of us who have lawns staked signs of gratitude. Most healthcare workers I spoke to, from cleaners to doctors, were uncomfortable with the word *hero*. Others were angry. They appreciated the kindness and support; some days, hearing the clanging pots and pans, or not having to worry about packing a lunch or finding an open take-out restaurant near the hospital was all that got them through the day. Vela joked that she was happy people finally realized there was more to the profession than fancy cars; doctors made sacrifices, too. She added that it was also humbling to see her community recognize the sacrifices she, and other frontline workers, made to work through the pandemic. It was their job, what they'd trained to do: they didn't need, or want, to be exalted. But it was also more complicated than that. Around the world, healthcare workers worried the hero worship made it too easy for governments to evade responsibility. In a healthcare system that worked and was well funded, they argued, heroic efforts would be unnecessary. There would be enough PPE, enough ventilators, enough safety.

"COVID-19 is not a terrorist or intergalactic villain," wrote one healthcare worker. "Heroes are not necessary to kill a virus. Heroes are a symptom that our system has failed." And that failure extended beyond the most visible front line, to another area where women largely made up the neglected troupes in charge of another life-saving measure: staying home.

"MOTHERING RIGHT NOW IS AN ESSENTIAL SERVICE."

Andrea O'Reilly,
York University professor

Five

CRISIS AT HOME

Natalie Bruvels knew it would be bad the moment professors ushered her class into a conference room. She doesn't remember the exact date her school announced the pandemic shutdown—everything that came after has blurred the early details, like tears splotched on a page, bleach on a stain. At thirty-nine, Bruvels was the only student in her master of fine arts program at the University of Ottawa with a young child. Speaking to the first- and second-year students nearing the end of their term, her professors tried to frame the campus closure as a boon. The positive spin presumed more time for creativity and research, a blessed pause from the daily grind. Those in the room collectively conjured images of blissful hours spent hunched over easels, masterpieces spun from fingertips, time to do the best work of their lives. Despite the fear and the uncertainty of the rapidly advancing virus, most people seemed determined to try the bright side. Given all that, Bruvels still can't believe what popped out of her mouth, as loud and clear and shocking as a gunshot: "I'm fucked."

March break was starting soon, and she'd been prepared to spend two weeks with her son, who is nine. But after that? She didn't believe his school would resume either. As a single mother, she didn't have another parent at home to help balance the weight of her new normal. Bruvels loved her art and her work but unlike the other students, on that last day on campus she didn't bother grabbing many supplies from the studio. She understood immediately that her painting practice was over, if only—hopefully—temporarily. She wanted to focus on keeping her son healthy, happy, stable; to do that along with all the work required for her master's felt impossible. At first, she did at least try to attend her online classes. But her overwhelmed son had an outburst every time, either during or after the class. Bruvels asked her professors if they could, perhaps, record their lectures so she could catch up in the evenings, after her son fell asleep. She was told everyone else had made the effort to attend class, so she should too. They were all in the same boat. Except, of course, they weren't.

"Something snapped in me at that point," she confessed. "I felt completely removed from my cohort." If her son could have her undivided attention, he seemed better able to cope with his inside-out world. Whenever she tried to multitask, though, he'd tailspin, angry. She kept asking herself, *How can this situation continue?* As it turned out, it didn't. After a few disastrous do-it-all attempts, she chose her son. The moment she mentally let go of school, Bruvels felt relief. As far as decisions went, this one was relatively easy—she hadn't had many other options. But she *had* chosen, and she could now feel that particular weight evaporate. Other decisions quickly rolled in to take its place. Unfortunately, parenting through a pandemic doesn't come with a manual. Nobody can tell you what to do when your usually sweet-natured kid becomes filled with sudden rage. For Bruvels, there were both good days and bad ones. Sometimes those days stitched together the good and bad moments, creating a tapestry of emotion and exhaustion. Bruvels and her son fell into a routine: every day they'd head to the empty greenbelt near their house and walk and talk, bush-whacking through the trees. Some days the hike would last an hour, other days they'd traipse for three. Bruvels remembers the beautiful scenery, the beautiful conversation, the beautiful reprieve. But one day in the forest was also the Worst Day.

Her son was mad at her for something. She thinks it was because they had gone for a walk in the forest, even though it was, at that point, their favourite thing to do. It gave them structure, routine, a way to decompress and talk about school, themselves, the virus—her son had taken to watching explainer videos about COVID-19 on YouTube. She hadn't expected this time to be any different, any less peaceful, magical. But her son, for whatever reason, did not want to be there that day. He began screaming at her, then charged her as though he was going to hit her. He didn't. But then he charged her again, this time barrelling his small body right into her. Bruvels was so startled she began to cry. Never, ever would she have expected her son to attack her. She had no idea how to deal with that type of violence and aggression from her kid. Nothing had prepared her for it, nothing had hinted that this would be a thing she'd need to know. *I know this is not my child*, she thought. *This is the madness of the world being funneled through him.* Even the good days often felt stressful. Homework was arduous, for both of them. Outside of the visits to the forest, she struggles to remember how she filled the rest of their days. They ate and they slept and they kept on trying to get through.

The Second Worst Day arrived in May. Bruvels was exhausted—a thing she feels almost silly saying. But she was, there was no escaping it, and one night she forgot about the hot water running into her bathtub. It overflowed, streaming through the light fixtures below, raining into her son's bedroom. He screamed that the house was collapsing. Bruvels ran to the bathroom, through the sloshing water, wrenching the tap. It was too late. The flood was catastrophic. Parts of the ceiling had buckled; pieces fell. The bathroom floor would have to be completely torn up, discarded. Later, when they needed something to laugh about, they joked that, because they couldn't travel, they brought Niagara Falls to them. Because that's what it had looked like: a rushing, deafening waterfall, sprung in their own house. Bruvels lives in a subsidized co-op, and they demanded she pay for the extensive repairs necessary to make the house liveable again. CERB, a school scholarship, and her paid job as a teaching assistant had given her a better cash flow than she'd had in years, but the idea of being able to afford the repairs still seemed laughable. There was just no way, and besides, her lease dictated she should be off the hook. So, Bruvels packed some clothes and other belongings for her and her son and moved in with her mother.

When I spoke to her months later in early August, she was still there, her own home a wreck. She'd had two weeks to work on her art while her son was in camp. She wanted nothing more than to continue to immerse herself in her school work, to paint, to feel the physicality of it, the empowerment, the joy. She felt frustrated, and maybe a little angry, that her professors and others were treating her as if, in asking for support and accommodations, she was looking for an easy way out. Taking stock of her life over the past few months, she knew nothing felt easy at all.

As provinces and territories began to close school doors in March, many parents—and particularly mothers—felt their days fracture. Unexpectedly and unwillingly they became math and English teachers, task managers, cafeteria cooks, classroom peacemakers, tech support, and home-school principals, all rolled into one ill-equipped package. Child care, already notoriously expensive and inaccessible, became obsolete. Mothers who worked at home were forced to teeter between staff Zoom calls, homework questions, meltdowns, work crises, laundry, lunch, the laughability of nine to five. Mothers who still worked outside the home were forced to make impossible decisions, beg favours, place heavy responsibility and the burden of grow-up-fast on their children, change shifts, quit jobs. Other mothers found themselves newly without income, navigating it all with one eye on their bank accounts.

Many parents, no matter their gender, felt the bruising pressure of the pandemic. There's no doubt fathers, and particularly single fathers, felt the pain, too. There's also little argument that, as is often the case, mothers felt it more. It should also be underscored that some mothers, including single mothers, racialized mothers, low-income mothers, and mothers parenting children with disabilities, experienced an even deeper strain. But few mothers had it easy. One in-depth May 2020 study by the U.K.-based Institute for Fiscal Studies (IFS) found that mothers were 23 per cent more likely than fathers to have lost their jobs during the pandemic. And, adding to the sting, mothers in the U.K. were also nearly 50 per cent more likely to have permanently lost employment, or to have quit. Throughout all this, they were looking after their children for an average of 10.3 hours every day, about 2.3 hours more than fathers. Mothers also, perhaps unsurprisingly, did about two hours more housework every day. If you're keeping track, that's twelve hours of non-paid work; now (try to) add to that a 7.5-hour workday, plus time to eat, sleep, go to the washroom, get dressed, breathe deeply, cry silently.

Then there's the labour that's more difficult to gauge in hours and percentage points: the emotional management of a home swiftly changed by worldwide trauma, illness, fear. Worrying about how to make everything all right when nothing is all right. Explaining to your four-year-old why they can't see their friends or hug their grandparents. Trying to reassure your ten-year-old that their grandparents won't die, even when you're anxious about that same thing, even when it seems like everyone might. Telling your sixteen-year-old they're not invincible, even though you desperately wish they were. Attempting to console your partner, live with their anger, love them, protect yourself, confront your constant proximity to each other. Wiping tears from chubby faces, properly oohing and aahing over Play-Doh masterpieces, gluing googly eyes, finding that one episode of that one show where the character does "the thing," chasing away nightmares, mediating sibling battles, baking the good cookies, giving a hug.

None of this work can be fully measured, not really, but there are ways in which we've tried. One couple working from home charted the number of interruptions from their eight- and twelve-year-old daughters on a random Thursday morning during lockdown. They later published the results in a *Washington Post* article: "The average length of an uninterrupted stretch of work time was three minutes, 24 seconds. The longest uninterrupted period was 19 minutes, 35 seconds. The shortest was mere seconds." They counted interruptions as anything intentional: requests for homework help, questions about chores and snacks, check-in hugs, tech support. Distractions, like "cello practice and shrieks of laughter," weren't included, but, the couple added, they did take their toll. And as the IFS noted, that toll was felt more often by mothers, who, on average, were only able to do one-third of the paid, uninterrupted work hours of fathers.

"Mothering right now is an essential service," York University professor Andrea O'Reilly told me several months into the pandemic. "Mothers are doing this work at a huge cost to their sanity, their leisure, their time, and their careers." O'Reilly has studied mothering for over three decades and has the c.v. to prove it: she is a professor at York's School of Gender, Sexuality, and Women's Studies, was the founder and director of the Motherhood Initiative for Research and Community Involvement from 1997–2020, and also the founder of Demeter Press, which publishes feminist work on mothering, reproduction, sexuality, and family. Which is all to say that while she was frustrated by the ways in which mothers were forgotten, unsupported, and failed during the pandemic, she wasn't exactly surprised. Like in so many other cases that exposed poor social support, the pandemic only magnified what was already there—a lack of good, affordable child care, a titled division of domestic labour, a seemingly impossible-to-breach wage gap. *This is not an equal-opportunity pandemic*, O'Reilly thought, watching it all unfold, her own children now adults. Whenever people said women were suffering more, she still liked to correct them. "Mothers are suffering more," she told people, "because they are the ones doing the care work."

O'Reilly felt galvanized to act against this normalization of so-called "women's work" after she stumbled across a post on

Facebook that detailed one single mother's experience in the Maritimes. The mom described being belittled and bullied at a Costco after being forced to take her young kids with her to get groceries, which was against the store's recommended rules. She needed supplies, most of her delivery had been cancelled because everything was out of stock, and the only person available to watch her four- and eight-year-old kids was her. She'd arrived at the store on April 2, tears streaming down her face after discovering she'd have to add home-schooling to the mix for who knows how long, only to have employee after employee berate her—as if she'd wanted to bring her kids to the store. It was the first time she'd left her house since the lockdown had begun weeks earlier. After reading the post, O'Reilly created a hashtag and splashed it everywhere she could, making an uncomfortable point: "#MothersAreFrontlineWorkers." Then she created a Facebook support group for mothers dealing with the pandemic. She wanted them to have a safe space to vent, to feel validated, to find resources; a place where they could say they were not okay and that, sometimes, neither were their kids. Within twenty-four hours, more than 250 moms had joined the group. By the time I spoke to O'Reilly a few months later, that number sat at 1,200.

Perhaps what most dismayed her, and many other mothers, was that, outside of their friend groups and Facebook pages, nobody seemed initially inclined to talk about the extra burden put on mothers. Not when governments shut down the economy, and not when they slowly started to reopen it before finding solutions for school and child care. The idea that moms will "take care of it"—whatever "it" may be, whether it's a scraped knee or a global pandemic—is deeply ingrained into our social psyche. Those in power seemed to assume women would, quite simply, figure it out. Too few were talking about how unsustainable it all was. In O'Reilly's Facebook group, mothers talked about having to look after kids and also their elderly, sometimes terminally ill, parents; about having to do all the cooking, while others in the family didn't recognize the energy it took; about being the only one relegated to washing every single fruit and vegetable before it went into the fridge; about falling behind at work; about guilt and children who felt neglected; and about mental and emotional breakdowns and their inevitability. One woman described it thus: "I hadn't realized marriage instantly meant that one person miraculously loses most of their cognitive functions and the other attains even more miraculous superpowers such as psychically knowing what is needed by every member of the household on two or four legs." Another said simply: "WTF just happened?"

Elsewhere, media slowly began to cover the domestic implosion—even if only to ask, as one late April *Today's Parent* article did, "Why is nobody talking about how unsustainable this is for working parents?" Some media cautioned of a "patriarchal pandemic" if governments didn't intercede to offer women more financial support and child care solutions—if, essentially, it didn't treat them like the essential workers O'Reilly, and eventually others, argued they were. *The Atlantic* got it right when it stated, early on, "The Coronavirus is a Disaster for Feminism." Enough with the arrogance and painful positivity, its author stated. Let's get real. Past pandemics foretold of everything that would come to pass: not only would women take the brunt of home responsibilities and lose out on work, they would feel these repercussions and distortions far into the future as men's income returned faster to pre-outbreak levels and more women spent more and more time caretaking. "All this looking after—this unpaid caring labor—will fall more heavily on women, because of the existing structure of the workforce," author Helen Lewis warned. She didn't exactly need a crystal ball, but for months the crisis buzzed underneath the news cycle, like background noise.

In June, the *New York Times* warned again that the "Pandemic Could Scar a Generation of Working Mothers." By July, it had declared, "In the COVID-19 Economy, You Can Have a Kid or Job. You Can't Have Both." The author, Deb Perelman, also bemoaned the muted alarm. "The consensus is that everyone agrees this is a catastrophe, but we are too bone-tired to raise our voices above a groan, let alone scream through a megaphone," she wrote. "Every single person confesses burnout, despair, feeling like they are losing their minds, knowing in their guts that this is untenable." Around that same time, a viral story emerged about one San Diego woman who'd been fired from her job because her boss could hear her young kids in the background on video calls. She decided to sue. For other women, the balance wasn't only untenable or unfair; it was also dangerous. Across the world, countries began to report rising domestic violence rates. In the U.K., suspected domestic homicides tripled during the first month of lockdown, with sixteen women and girls murdered. In Canada, domestic violence workers noted a surge in both the prevalence and severity of violence. Women reported that their abusers used the isolation of the pandemic to increase control, bending information about both the rules and the virus to limit their ability to seek help. Others legitimately feared increased contact at a shelter. Plans to leave abusive situations were abruptly curtailed. Many shelters found themselves in urgent need of new volunteers. "When COVID-19 hit back in March we scaled up our crisis line to be 24/7," said Angela Marie MacDougall, executive director of B.C.-based Battered Women's Support Services, at the end of August. "Since then, calls to our crisis line have increased by up to 300 per cent." She needed another twenty new volunteers to keep up with all the calls. For far too many women, nowhere felt comfortable. Nowhere felt safe.

For many pregnant mothers, the hospital seemed like the scariest place of all. Tali Bogler is a physician and the chair of family medicine obstetrics at St. Michael's Hospital in Toronto. In March, her twin daughters were not quite three years old; she didn't have to reach back to remember her own pregnancy anxiety. And that was in normal times. When the pandemic was declared, it felt to Bogler like a huge, invisible switch had flipped. Even though she hadn't closed her practice, her phone began ringing cancellation after cancellation. Pregnant women left her office with tears pelting down their faces. Others phoned ahead to ask if they should come into their appointment, shocked and unsure of what to do. Every common worry had ballooned in size, and then burst. Bogler understood their *pop! pop! pop!* of fear. Her first thought when the WHO declared the pandemic was, *How am I going to support women during this time?*

But she, like everyone else, had few answers about how hazardous the virus was to pregnant people. Her mind went to the Zika virus, which the WHO named a global health emergency in 2016. At the time, the health agency warned pregnant women, or those who might become pregnant, not to travel to nearly one hundred countries and regions. If a child-bearing person became infected, the virus could damage the fetal nervous system, even if said person didn't develop symptoms. If that damage did occur, the baby could develop congenital Zika syndrome, which has five key markers, including brain damage. The Canadian federal government had lifted travel warnings related to Zika only a few months earlier. Initially, Bogler had no way of knowing if COVID-19 would pose a similar threat or become something even worse. Viruses in general tended to attack the immunocompromised, and both pregnant people and newborns fit into that category. (It's worth noting that, six months into the pandemic, information on how the virus affects pregnant people and newborns remained distressingly deficient; some early data has shown that pregnant people are more at risk and are 70 per cent more likely to need respirators if they do get the virus, but a Grand Canyon of questions has persisted.)

Even if the new coronavirus spared them, Bogler knew that the mass shutdown of services would affect her patients in other, detrimental ways. "It was such a shock for pregnant women, because you do everything you can to have a healthy pregnancy," she said. You eat the right foods, sign up for the right classes, avoid all the risks. "And then this was something completely out of control for them." Women who had the resources for prenatal classes were abruptly left with nothing. Grandparents who had intended to be present for the baby's birth or to provide support in the postpartum period were forced to stay home. Community supports were nullified. Women who were already facing higher risks only saw them skyrocket. Add to all that the absolute paralyzing fear of not knowing if your newborn could catch COVID-19, or what it would do to them if they did. And add to that the destabilizing uncertainty of bringing a new life into a world throttled by a pandemic. A world that nobody thought would ever be the same again. There was no "ultimate guide" for that.

Within days of receiving the lockdown orders, Bogler and other providers she worked with began to brainstorm new ways they could reassure—and reach—their patients. They landed on a simple, but highly effective, solution: Instagram. Not only was it free and easily accessible, but they knew that many pregnant people fit into the platform's demographic. In early April, they launched an account under the name Pandemic Pregnancy Guide, and gave the page a cheeky description: "What to expect when you're expecting . . . during a pandemic." The colour scheme is a checkerboard of Insta-calm, all rich teal and blush pink. The tone of each post exhibits the same calm; captions are evidence-based, competent, clear. Early posts talked about whether patients in labour were wearing masks; how prenatal care might change; the likelihood of hospitals reducing the "one support person" rule to zero, a controversial and panic-producing move that would force people to give birth alone. Comments were both anxious and thankful, vacillating between posters who expressed general alarm and those who, in typical Insta fashion, thanked organizers, left heart emojis, and said things like "bless."

Bogler and the other founders expected their followers would include their immediate patients, and maybe their friends. Instead, the page quickly gained more than ten thousand followers. As their numbers and profile grew, the team started to receive sponsorship offers. Bogler turned them all down. It was important for her that the information remain free from influence and bias; the information is strictly medical and that's it. By September 2020, the page had hosted dozens of live expert sessions, on everything from optimal birth positions to going to the ER during the initial outbreak surge. As the country began to reopen schools, the account also addressed the extra anxieties of families with school-aged kids. They hosted a Pride-themed prenatal and postpartum workout, and they discussed intimate partner violence. They talked about Black maternal health, diversified their experts, and even tackled post-pregnancy sex. In a time particularly rife with social media and "I heard that . . ." misinformation, Bogler and her colleagues worked hard to quell uncertainty and provide good information. They listened to feedback about the platform and got better at all the tech stuff and savvy branding. "None of us are influencers on Instagram," said Bogler. "We're all learning things as we go."

Across the country in Vancouver, Nusha Balram was also learning as she went. On March 1, 2020, she had officially gone on maternity leave from her job at a trade union, where she works in human rights and equity training. About a month before that, a pregnant Balram, her nine-year-old son, her mother, and her partner had moved out of the 65-square-metre attic apartment they all shared and into a space with a backyard big enough to build a tree house. "Oh my God," they all joked, "look, we're all hanging out in the same room and we're not even touching!" It was perfect. And then, just a few weeks later on March 13, the city went into lockdown. Within days, she realized how bad everything might get—how different it would all be—when she looked at her bank account. Everything was refunded: her mom-and-baby yoga classes, all their upcoming community centre programs, the summer YMCA camp for her son. She had three thousand dollars of cancelled spring and summer plans sitting there in dollar signs and zeros. Then, her midwife team announced they were switching to phone-only appointments. Before then, she'd visited the duo every two weeks, sometimes every week. They were friends with her and her partner. Suddenly, she couldn't see them at all.

"I felt a little lost," said Balram. It was hard for her to figure out her next best steps because every day felt like a different reality. The case numbers kept changing, and with them the recommendations for what to do, how to keep safe. Every single day, Balram stayed glued to her TV, waiting for Dr. Bonnie Henry's daily announcement, a small compass in the chaos: "Everybody knows Dr. Henry is the best." Some days, it felt like the stay-at-home order was just issued yesterday; other days it felt like they'd been self-quarantining for years. Every day was the same, and every day was built on a foundation of anxiety. Balram was exhausted, very pregnant, and hadn't yet decided where she would give birth. Before the lockdown, she and her partner had been negotiating whether to go to the hospital or stay home. Her partner, who is Indigenous, felt strongly about a home birth; he'd wanted to honour traditional practices, such as smudging and drumming. Balram was more on the fence. She'd given birth to her son, who has a different father, at the B.C. Women's Hospital, and remembered the experience as "wonderful." And as COVID-19 descended on her city, she began to feel guilty about asking her doula and midwife team to forgo the safety of the hospital.

Balram had plenty of time to think about it during her near week of non-progressive contractions. With nowhere to go, she'd sit on her roof deck all day, watching the sluggish tempo of the new world below. And then, in the middle of the night, after everyone agreed to try a home birth, she finally went into labour. Her doula arrived at the house at 5 a.m., dressed in full PPE. The midwife team arrived shortly after that, also in full safety armor. Balram hardly noticed what they were wearing at all. It was an excruciating, difficult, lovely birth. Balram was one of the roughly 25 per cent of women to experience back labour, which is exceptionally gruelling and is usually caused when the baby is facing the stomach instead of the spine. There wasn't much she could do at home to ease the agony besides get in the bath, which she didn't want to do. Without an epidural, or other hospital-only treatments, she needed her big support team to get her through the pain; they all had a job, or three. A kind word. Encouragement. Back massage. Water. Distraction. Helping her to switch positions. At last, at about 8 a.m., her daughter was born. It was April 20, "which will probably be annoying for me when she's a teenager," joked Balram. Somebody took a cute picture of the midwives in full PPE, giving little peace signs. Under the mask, goggles, and cap, you can't see their smiling faces at all.

The next day, over Facetime from Saskatchewan, her partner's parents sang the warrior song to their new grandchild.

It was meant to help her be strong. It was also meant to be sung as soon as the baby was born, the first words she heard. But COVID-19 had forced the excited to-be grandparents to cancel their initial plans to fly out for the birth. It was still a sweet moment, but it wasn't the same. There were a lot of things that weren't the same. When Balram was pregnant with her son, she worked at a settlement agency, often organizing multicultural pot luck lunches for the forty or so diverse seniors under her care. After she gave birth, she brought her son out to one of those lunches, where he was passed around, cuddled and kissed, tickled and held. It was, as Balram put it, "basically like having forty grandmas and grandpas." This time, there was no bubbling joy that accompanied introducing her new child to loved ones, friends, acquaintances. Her girlfriends couldn't drop by her new place to marvel over her daughter's tiny curled fists, her soft skin and precious face. Even when it became safe to meet for a socially distanced lunch outside, nobody could hold her daughter but her. When her daughter cried, or if Balram just needed a break, she just had to keep on holding her. It was weird and sad and more than a little heartbreaking.

"It's been this constant swing of emotion," said Balram. "The theme of this entire time is feeling a lot of loss, but also feeling a lot of privilege." Even in the darkness, she had much to cherish. Her daughter was healthy and safe, and so too were the rest of her family. Co-parenting her son wasn't easy even before the pandemic, but she felt grateful his father took the outbreak as seriously as she did. Honestly, thinking about her past relationship with her ex, she felt grateful she wasn't isolating in the house with him, stuck in something that didn't work. She felt really grateful that she'd been able to move before the lockdown and was no longer in the tiny, impossible space where she knew she'd have figuratively killed somebody, probably even before self-isolation. As it turned out, her partner and her kid did build a treehouse in the new backyard, and it was beautiful. Her son learned to cook. She felt privileged to have her mat leave, to be able to spend so much time with her family. She was even thankful she got to be there for the tough stuff, like taking her son to the city's Juneteenth protests at the height of that spring's Black Lives Matter activism. They talked about what it meant to be people of colour, what it meant to be Indigenous, what it meant to be Black. They talked about colonialism and racism and injustice.

But perhaps the best moment of all came in July when her partner's parents, having had no cases at all in the town where they live, decided it was safe to make the trek to visit their son and his family. When they arrived, they sang the warrior song in person, and they held their granddaughter—the first new people outside of her own household and the midwives to do so since she was born, nearly three months before.

Mandi Freeman didn't want to quit her job. She'd tried running a home daycare; she'd tried hosting Tupperware parties; she'd tried online entrepreneurship. She'd tried just about everything, and loved none of it. But this job was different.

In December 2019, she'd started work as a home care aide—
her first full-time gig after more than a decade of mothering
her five kids. It immediately clicked. The days were long and
often hard, spent bouncing around Cranbrook, B.C., in and
out of clients' homes from morning to night. She was good at
it, though. Clients told her she brought something special
to the job, and Freeman felt it too: she'd found her purpose.
"I was damn good at my job," she recalled. "This was it for me."
She'd always wanted to help people, and now she could see
the difference she made in their lives every day. Plus, she was
in a good groove. She had energy, a schedule, a meal prepping
system, and she was wearing clothes that were neither pyjamas
nor tank tops stained and stretched from nursing. She was
being herself, finding her identity. Things were going so great
that she'd planned to attend school in September 2020 to get
accredited. Then, over the course of January and February,
she became the sickest she'd ever been in her life.

Today, Freeman is convinced she had COVID-19, probably
caught from one of her clients. Officially, she has no answers.
Whatever it was, doctors misdiagnosed it as pneumonia three
times. No antibiotic seemed to help. At one point, she was put
on doxycycline, a powerful drug that treats a variety of serious bugs and that, in this case, left Freeman with a nasty side
effect—permanent acid reflux disease. The illness cascaded
through her house, and soon everybody was sick. It took most
of February for them all to recover and go back to school and
work. A couple of weeks later, the world declared a pandemic.

Freeman's children are all under the age of twelve. The oldest is eleven and the youngest is three. Her partner's job at a metal fabrication plant was deemed essential. So too was Freeman's. It hardly mattered. With no school and no child care, she didn't see how they could both possibly continue working full-time. Now, she thinks of her gut reaction as selfish; there was a lot more at stake than her job. At the time, though, all she could think was: *How am I going to keep working?* She was— rightfully—angry at the virus for interrupting her budding career. That anger blanketed her emotions, turning to numbness. Leaving her new job felt inevitable, no matter what angle Freeman examined the problem from.

After schools confirmed classes would resume online following March break, Freeman knew she'd have to phase herself out of her job in April. During a pandemic, however, that was easier said than done; demand for home help was high and desperate. Freeman told her employer she could only work three hours a day. In return, her supervisor asked if she could get someone down the street to look after her children— a move that would, of course, break lockdown rules. At first, her work commitment only increased; she worked thirty-seven days with no break. Freeman stuck to her guns, though, and slowly, regretfully began to reduce both her client numbers and hours. In the Before Times, she'd work from 9 a.m. to 4 p.m., sometimes longer, and come home for a break or two in between clients. In COVID Times, she equipped her oldest daughter with a cellphone and left her in charge after breakfast.

Her significantly cut hours also meant she wouldn't be out of their house for too long. Freeman said she often justified it to herself: they were okay, the client's house was only a few minutes away, she wasn't leaving town, the children had eaten breakfast and started their school work. Everything was *fine.* "Yeah," she said, "that didn't last long either."

In June, she'd emailed her boss to say that she'd need a leave of absence. Her husband had, at that point, been laid off and could stay with the kids. It was all breaking down, anyway. She felt filled and overflowing with guilt, anxiety. There was too much screen time for her kids; some of them were struggling with school. Her eldest daughter was having constant night-mares that her friends were contracting COVID and dying. When her partner was still working, she felt like she was in survival mode: *If you want to eat seven granola bars, sure, just have an apple somewhere in between. Twenty minutes of schoolwork is enough, congratulations. Can I go to the bath-room alone, please?* They were spending more than they could afford on fast food because everybody was too sad and too tired to cook. Even after her partner was forced home to help, the exhaustion continued. Her kids were crying all the time; she was crying all the time. They hadn't seen their friends in ages; she hadn't seen her friends in ages. Nobody was sleeping properly. Freeman felt stuck, and she knew her family did, too. "From mid-March to the May long weekend," she said, "was hell and depression and darkness and too much TV and laziness."

While she'd been loath to quit her job at first, in the end it felt like taking back her power—grabbing some control in the chaos. She knew her energy would be better spent at home; she needed to hold on to her kids, both literally and figuratively. She also wanted to be home so she could talk to them about what was happening, guide them through the pandemic. Freeman knew the self-quarantine months would feel like a defining moment of their childhood once they were adults. She wanted them to come out of it as unscathed as possible. To do any of that, she needed to be present. And to help explain the pandemic and the skewed world it created, the way that everything had changed, she needed to first take the time to explain it to herself. She needed to pause, process, and herself grasp what the heck was going on. To her, trying to explain and soothe while lost in a bog of stress and misinformation felt impossible. "I think," she joked, "I can talk about sex more comfortably with them than the pandemic." At least with sex, there were books, facts, shows, finite knowledge; she'd experienced it herself. "But to talk to them about surviving a pandemic and what their lives are going to look like afterwards—I don't have those answers yet."

She decided to do something radical to interrupt the fear. Freeman loaded up as much as she could fit into her motor home and drove her family out to the bush—no place special in particular. As she put it: you don't have to drive far from Cranbrook in any direction to hit a dirt road, and then you keep going until you find a creek or a lake. Out there, she helped the kids keep up with school work as much as she could, but mostly she put her emphasis on a different kind of education: safety, comfort, love. Her youngest learned how to swim. Her oldest learned how to read maps. All that bubbling stress began to leak out, evaporate. Soon, her kids were calling it The Best Summer Ever. To Freeman, it wasn't throwing in the towel so much as it was choosing how her family could best make it through. Frankly, living in the motor home was also drastically cheaper—a big plus after Freeman resigned and stopped driving into town every day for her shifts. Having lost his job, her partner was relying on employment insurance (EI), and once she later went on leave, Freeman's income was reduced to CERB. In the bush, she wasn't buying fast food, running showers and baths for seven people, doing endless loads of dishes and laundry. Even in the summer, her hydro bill was $150 every month; now it was $9.

And if she sometimes missed her budding career, and dreaded thinking about September, well, she hoped things happened for a reason. "I can see that I'm going to look back at our time in the bush ten years from now and think, 'Damn, this is exactly what I needed,'" she said. "This is exactly what my children needed."

"OH MY GOD. WHAT AM I GOING TO DO?"

Alèthe Kaboré,
entrepreneur

Six

THE SHE-CESSION

Alèthe Kaboré had planned 2020 down to the last loonie. In October 2019, she'd officially launched her dream business, KYN Apparel, with a splashy runway show in Calgary. Watching the models strut the spotlight wearing her designs—Canadian-weather cuts mixed with bold African prints—had given her the best feeling ever. It had been a risk to start her business and follow a passion so far outside her formal education, but now she allowed herself to think it would pay off. The business loan, tumbling into debt, putting herself out there, everything else she had done to get where she was—it might just work out after all. Kaboré had moved to Edmonton in 2006 from Burkina Faso to study biological sciences at university. Later on, she earned a master of science in public health. Since graduating, though, she had struggled to find permanent work in her field and had been thinking a lot in 2019 about what else she could do—if it was worth it to take the leap. Not seeing many other Black, immigrant women in Alberta's fashion industry, and having few mentors who looked like her, had caused her to doubt herself more than once. It didn't help that ever since she was a kid growing up in Burkina Faso, she, like most of her peers, had planned to study science, pursue a stable career, become a doctor or a researcher. "Everybody's kind of going the same direction," she said, of the persistent doubt. "And you're trying to go in a different one."

Kaboré had always adored fashion, but she didn't learn to sew until shortly after moving to Alberta, at which point she began to teach herself. She had missed the colourful and vibrant clothes of her birth country and, unable to find anything like them where she now lived, decided to make her own. At first, whenever she wore dresses and blouses with African patterns to school and work, people would ask her if she was heading out to a party after; baffled, she'd respond, "No, this is what I usually wear." Kaboré wasn't about to ditch her bright aesthetic, but the ignorant comments got her thinking. She began to imagine a fusion of office wear and African style, and also started experimenting with merging the sunny, dynamic fabric that felt like home with designs that better matched Canada's frigid climate. Pretty soon, she'd show up to places and people would beg her to make them one of whatever she was wearing. Their reactions gave her the confidence to start taking clothing samples to community events and African Fashion Week shows. The enthusiasm she received there, in turn, built the confidence she needed to try making her budding business her full-time job. People kept asking her for expanded styles, added sizes. They kept saying, *more*. After the October kickoff, Kaboré got another major boost. In early 2020, she won the African Fashion and Arts Movement's designer of the year award. *Okay*, she thought, *I can do this. There's hope there.*

Over the next few months, Kaboré cemented her expansion plans. She booked fashion shows across the country, filling in the entire calendar year. She snapped up bundles of fabric and began growing her inventory. She even hired another seamstress to help meet demand and took first steps toward finding manufacturers in China. Closer to home, she signed up for a booth at the local farmers' market, determined to bring both her culture and her style into the usually homogeneous space. She put out press releases and began to connect with others in her community. She had a strategy to drive traffic to her website, to transition out of her day job in 2021, and to begin paying herself a salary from her business by the end of the year. She would pay back her small business loan months ahead of time. By March, her ducks were in a neat, ambitious row, and Kaboré was excited about the months ahead. "And then, everything happened," she said. "I was like, 'Oh my God. What am I going to do?'" Initially, she allowed herself to believe it would be a momentary setback—a month at most—and then reality would reassert itself. A month hadn't passed, though, before all her carefully booked events began to cancel. "And now I'm just freaking out," she said. The world had scrubbed a giant-sized eraser over her plans.

She had extra machines, fabric, supplies, and enough clothes to take to her next several scheduled shows and stock her website. She had bills. At least she also still had her job at the library. As that moved to work-from-home, however, Kaboré's space started to feel decidedly un-Marie-Kondo-like. Both her home office and her home inventory had to be shoved inside one space. She was often physically in the middle, trying to traverse through—a metaphor for her possible career paths, frustrations, and fears brought to life. Kaboré's first step, after the shock, was to try and cater to demand. Drawing on her public health expertise, she started sewing cheerful face masks and selling them on the KYN Apparel website. It helped bring in sales, but not as much cash flow as she needed. She reluctantly explored further loan options, but—at least intially— ultimately decided she didn't want to become one of the many small businesses that sank further into the red during the pandemic. In July, the Canadian Federation of Independent Business (CFIB) estimated that three-quarters of small businesses had taken on extra debt to keep afloat, totalling a depressing $117 billion. On average, each business added $135,000 to its debt, with business owners relying on personal savings, credit cards, bank loans, and retirement savings (in that order). By mid-September, only 18 per cent of businesses in Alberta were at or above normal revenues, though 65 per cent of them had reopened.

Even if she had decided to incur more debt during the early months of the pandemic, Kaboré isn't sure she would have been successful at doing so. She didn't have much luck finding grants or other funding, either, despite dedicated searching.

There just wasn't anything out there—or if there was, she didn't have access to it. "In the business world, there is segregation," she said. "The men are getting the most of the pie, and when it comes to women, the white women are getting more than the Black women." (In fact, in recognition of this, Justin Trudeau announced a $221 million funding program in September 2020 to help Black business owners and entrepreneurs access funding and capital, as well as loans and other services.) Kaboré also worried that closing her business would be the equivalent of staking a flashing neon WARNING! sign, complete with not-so-fine print: Don't Try. How many other Black women who'd been thinking about starting a business would see that she'd shut down and decide not to take the risk themselves? She worried the answer might be "a lot," and that unknowable number weighed on her. She knew failure wasn't singular; it rippled out. But planning seemed impossible when the future was edged in ambiguity. The only thing she could do, she decided, was take it day by day—and hope the pandemic would fade before she tripped over the precipice.

Saschie MacLean-Magbanua dreamed people would miss her studio so much that when she reopened in June they'd rush back, ready to dance away the pandemic stress. That isn't exactly what happened. Her first month back at Formation, the ultra-cool white-and-concrete space she'd opened in Vancouver's Mount Pleasant neighbourhood at the end of 2019, was quiet. In part, that was because she'd reduced her

230-square-metre studio capacity by 65 per cent to help keep people safe. Instead of the thirty-five classes a week she ran in March—drawing up to a total of eight hundred people—she was now holding between fifteen and seventeen hours of class. But MacLean-Magbanua knew it wasn't the only reason her once-bustling studio felt subdued. Many people didn't yet feel comfortable sweating and shouting next to others, no matter the social distance. Some didn't feel comfortable leaving their house. Others likely could no longer afford the class. Or maybe they didn't know Formation had reopened. It didn't help that MacLean-Magbanua had chosen her location to draw in commuters and office folk, a move that felt like a score when there were still offices open for people to go to. Now the city was eerily empty, foot traffic defeated to zilch. She'd seen her class numbers rise each week, but still wondered if the trickle would be enough to sustain the business she'd poured her heart into.

MacLean-Magbanua hadn't always planned to open a dance studio; she isn't a dancer by training. But in 2014, her seventeen-year-old younger sister was in a fatal car accident, mere weeks before MacLean-Magbanua's twenty-sixth birthday. Shocked with grief, she retreated into herself. She spent weeks on her couch, watching-but-not-watching endless seasons of *Grey's Anatomy*, eating barbecue chips, quiet and still. During this time, MacLean-Magbanua was also seeing a grief counsellor who, one day, suggested she try moving her body every now and then, if she could. It would be good for her, the therapist coaxed. It might help her find some balance through the instability of loss. So when she saw a friend announce on Instagram that he was teaching an all-Beyoncé dance class, she decided to go. She was immediately surprised by the joy it gave her. The empowering, badass beats, moving to the choreography—it all helped to give her a welcome break from her own head. Her then-boyfriend, and now husband and business partner, suggested that she organize her own casual class, just her and a few friends having a blast and dancing to nothing but Beyoncé songs. MacLean-Magbanua was eager to revisit the sense of peace she had found through dance. She announced a drop-in class, expecting a few friends who felt obligated to come. Instead, the class was over capacity. "And it really snowballed from there," she said.

For the next few years, she ran drop-in classes three times a week in Vancouver, and hosted pop-ups in Calgary and Toronto under the name RSVP 33. Many of the people who attended the class were beginner dancers, or hadn't stepped into a studio since they were kids. MacLean-Magbanua welcomed all levels of experience. For her, the classes' ethos wasn't so much about perfecting the moves—although clients certainly learned new skills—but about providing a space where people could feel empowered, silly, sexy, or whatever else they needed to feel in that particular moment. She wanted them to feel safe enough, and supported enough, to unlock something in their bodies: grief, trauma, happiness, loss. She wanted them to have fun. Throughout RSVP 33's rapid organic growth, she kept her day job in tourism communications and marketing, working full-time right up until she decided to open a permanent studio and rebrand as Formation. By February, her new business had started to hit its groove. She was looking forward to March. Within a week of the month's start, however, an uneasy, anxious feeling thrummed through the city. MacLean-Magbanua remembers looking at the studio's schedule on Wednesday, March 11. Every day straight through Monday was booked solid. And then on Friday, Saturday, and Sunday, more people started dropping off, one by one, leaves in autumn. On Monday, March 16, MacLean-Magbanua ran her usual 7 a.m. class, not yet knowing it would be the last one.

After the class, she and her husband went out for coffee to chat about what they should do. Everything felt eerie and possibly unsafe. Their province hadn't yet announced a state of emergency, but neither one wanted to put their employees or their clients in danger. They'd stocked the studio with hand sanitizer and encouraged people to wash their hands. But nobody could tell them if they had done enough because nobody knew. Like many others, they felt stuck in limbo, collecting more questions than answers. And so, that morning, they decided to shut down the studio. It felt wrong to keep it open, pretending there was no risk. MacLean-Magbanua felt relieved to have finally made a decision, and it also broke her heart. She had no idea if she'd scrape together enough cash to keep paying rent. Her team didn't qualify for EI because they hadn't been open long enough, and at the time, they had no idea if extra aid was coming—or if their employees would qualify for it. When she locked the doors that day, she didn't know when, or if, she'd ever reopen them again for her clients. "Truthfully, the future is unclear for us," she wrote in a graceful Instagram post announcing the closure. "This is not a time to panic, it is a time for us all to take responsibility, stay grounded, and do our part."

For the first few weeks of the lockdown, MacLean-Magbanua was, as she puts it, "an emotional disaster." Everything that was spinning around the world—the shock, trauma, grief—was also a tornado inside of her, every bad headline a new piece of debris. But in between journalling and becoming a *Bon Appétit* superfan, MacLean-Magbanua was also working hard to help her business make it through. Like many fitness studio owners, she and her husband crafted a plan to try online classes. They had already invested in film equipment and, after brief inertia, moved quickly to film their instructors inside the studio, creating a vault of footage; luckily, the space was big enough to do it safely. In addition to building a digital content library, MacLean-Magbanua also chose to offer regular free live video classes, something she kept up for months, including after reopening in June. She wanted her instructors to have an opportunity to work. She also figured people just needed to dance. She didn't want to hoard such a powerful healing tool, one that had anchored her when she thought it was impossible. "Even if you're not in the same room, you're collectively creating energy for your space," she said. "It was like we were all still together." And, in a time of crushing isolation, that counted for a lot.

By far her biggest emotional challenge was not worrying what would happen to Formation itself, but what would happen to her team. MacLean-Magbanua had the foresight to make her instructors staff employees, not contractors, unlike many in the fitness industry—meaning, they'd be eligible for support they otherwise might not have received. In the early chaotic days, though, that support was like having a wish without a genie's lamp. She felt an overwhelming, suffocating responsibility right up until the start of CERB, which she and her husband also accessed. Relief for her business didn't come until much later. When it was first launched on April 9, the Canada Emergency Business Account (CEBA) program had an applicant threshold of $50,000 in payroll in 2019. As a new business, MacLean-Magbanua couldn't meet it. When it later dropped to $25,000, she was finally able to access the interest-free loan program, which offers small businesses and non-profits up to $40,000. By October 2020, more than 750,000 businesses had received CEBA loans, totalling $30.24 billion. A $5,000 grant from Bumble (yes, the dating app) had kept MacLean-Magbanua going until then. She felt fortunate for the cash, even if, in June, she still wasn't sure what her future held.

Already, many fellow business owners in her network had made the difficult decision to close permanently. Driving down the street where Formation is located, she'd see a checker-board of dark storefronts. Each one was a lost livelihood, a vanished community, the culmination of someone's hustle and hard work and creativity suddenly gone. She sometimes wondered if she would join them.

Spring 2020 wasn't all shuttered windows and red ink: threaded through all the loss and hardship, business owners found jewels of community, generosity, and ingenuity. Some also found belonging. Along with her husband and their three children, Sarah Taher moved to Fredericton, New Brunswick, from Dubai at the end of June 2019. The family is Muslim and originally from Egypt; they left both places because, as Taher put it, "We wanted a place we can call home." The family applied to move to Canada under New Brunswick's immigration pro-gram—although, Taher admitted, she had never before heard of the province itself. It wasn't a happy welcoming. Really, she didn't feel welcome at all. Fredericton's lack of racial and cul-tural diversity shocked her; it felt like she had arrived on a completely different planet. (The 2016 census shows that vis-ible minorities comprise less than 10 per cent of Fredericton's population.) She felt like she, and her hijab, had popped the Maritime town's white, isolated bubble. The only friends she was able to make were other Egyptian immigrants, other people who looked just like her. One of them apologetically told her, "Don't try to be friends with Canadians. They will never like you." A man in the supermarket yelled right in her face, "Ignorant mountain girl!" She thought: *What is that?* She thought: *Will I ever fit in?* She was depressed and lonely, an outsider in the place she wanted to call home.

Both Taher and her husband are engineers. After her arrival in Canada, Taher eventually got a job working from home as an SEO specialist for a Toronto-based company. She enjoyed it, but she had always wanted to start her own business. An idea for what it could be had started forming even before she moved to Canada: she wore custom-made hijabs; she could make beautiful, unique head coverings for others, too. She'd always wanted to learn how to sew and had vowed to cross it off her bucket list after moving to Fredericton. As she planned her new business and dodged closed-minded attitudes, she also started taking sewing lessons, watching online tutorials, and practising with her own machine and materials. In January, she felt skilled enough to open her own business, Sufeya, selling handmade scrunchies and hijabs both online and in person at the city's Northside Market. There, she finally started to feel like she was part of something. A florist at a nearby booth helped Taher on her first day, showed her to her table, and kindly and patiently answered all of her questions. Taher had also started a blog to process and share her experiences with discrimination in Canada. Readers started to visit her, buying silky, colourful hijabs—even if they weren't Muslim, even if they never planned to wear them.

Two months later, COVID-19 couldn't interrupt Taher's burgeoning sense of community. In fact, against all odds, it accelerated its progress. Forced away from the market, Taher, like Kaboré, looked at her leftover cotton material and decided to begin making masks. She was surprised when they were an immediate hit. "I've sold hundreds," she told me in July, just a few weeks after her one-year anniversary in Canada. "I've stopped counting, actually." She'd wake up early, spend a couple of hours making masks, work a six-hour shift for her day job, then spend time with her family. She dedicated most of her weekends to sewing, finishing one mask every ten minutes—she could now probably do it blindfolded, she joked. While she shipped her masks all over the country, she also sold plenty locally, both directly to customers and through local vendors. Working with the latter to buy fabric supplies, sell her finished product, and coordinate prize giveaways only widened her network. Her husband often delivered the masks himself, driving around Fredericton, dropping them off and saying hello. "I started to actually like the place," she said. "I thought, 'I can be part of this. People are starting to give me a chance. They're getting to know me.'" In the middle of a pandemic, both sides were starting to build trust.

This kind of community echoed throughout the country. People encouraged each other to buy local, to order every week from their favourite restaurants, to purchase monthly passes and yearlong memberships to small gyms and studios that they couldn't go to. In return, many restaurants and other shops donated food and supplies to frontline efforts, to homeless populations, to anyone who needed it. Thousands joined Taher, Kaboré, and MacLean-Magbanua in getting creative and pivoting their business, whether by adopting new practices, making entirely new products, or both. Plenty of designers started crafting masks. Distilleries began making hand sanitizer. Restaurants assembled meal kits and picnic baskets. Gyms and fitness studios across Canada moved their classes online and into living rooms. Consultants, instructors, and therapists alike offered video sessions. Musicians streamed concerts. Indeed, on the whole, women-owned businesses were more likely to enact changes during the initial months of the pandemic. Over half of them introduced new ways to interact with or sell to customers. And more than one-third modified their products or services—compared to just over one-quarter of all businesses in Canada. In other words: they got creative so they could survive.

Unfortunately, in many cases, it simply wasn't enough. In Toronto, seventy-seven-year-old Frances Wood was one of the many restaurant owners to call it quits. After nearly forty years, she closed her famous Cajun-and-Creole spot, Southern Accent, in April, which had served everyone from Helen Mirren to the Rolling Stones. The closure curtailed several decades' worth of plans to sell the restaurant and use the profit for her retirement; she told media that her future "doesn't look good." By the end of June, about 40 per cent of women-owned businesses were forced to lay off employees, and more than 30 per cent had to reduce staff hours. What's more, nearly two-thirds of those who did lay off workers sent pink slips to 80 per cent of their staff. Women also account for almost 40 per cent of self-employed Canadians; many of them rely on contractors, not employees, to run their business. Both factors put the majority of government support programs out of their reach (something that was true even before the pandemic). On top of that, small and medium-sized enterprises with under twenty employees—the type of business women are more likely to own—suffered disproportionately more revenue loss than larger companies with over one hundred employees. More women business owners reported being unable to pay their rent or mortgage payments, and more women reported being denied payment deferrals. In other words, while many businesses and entrepreneurs buckled under the mass shutdowns, for women the economic story was gloomier and more complicated.

That's largely because the crisis only heightened barriers women already face in the business world: a lack of access to capital, a bias against the sectors where they're most represented, and unbalanced domestic responsibilities. In April, the Canadian Women's Chamber of Commerce and the Dream Legacy Foundation teamed up to survey underrepresented founders and entrepreneurs about the impacts of the economic shutdown on their business, home life, and mental health. It defined underrepresented as "those outside the main entrepreneurship narrative"—i.e., anyone who wasn't white, cisgender-male, or Canadian-born. The results are depressing. While data showed that only 22 per cent of small businesses in Canada expected a 10 to 20 per cent decrease in revenue at the time, a whopping 50 per cent of those surveyed reported the same. More than 60 per cent of women-owned businesses stated they had lost contracts, customers, or clients, compared to 34 per cent of all small businesses in Canada. More than half told of negative health impacts and roughly the same number said they'd taken on additional child care duties. When narrowed down to racialized respondents' experiences, the already-dismal numbers worsened. A full 80 per cent of racialized founders of all genders reported lost contracts, customers, or clients. It's perhaps no wonder that their mental health costs were similarly higher.

One Indigenous woman in B.C. shared her experience: "I am home trying to balance work and family life. My sales have dropped significantly and I am facing delays in the shipping of my supplies and my product. I am limited to pursue my growth plans as they involved travel to the U.S. I have had to defer several bills due to no revenue coming in from sales." A Black businessowner in Montreal wrote of not receiving refunds for cancelled events, adding that all of her funding applications had been unceremoniously cancelled. A facilitator in St. John's chillingly noted that nobody was interested in training because they didn't know if they would be around in a year. Others reported not being able to take meetings and important business calls because they were parenting their children. Many had lost revenue from long-term, almost-completed projects that were abruptly trashed.

Event and conference revenue vanished. One woman in Whitehorse summed up the strange reverse feeling of sixty-to-zero: "Within one week, we lost every single booked contract we had for the foreseeable future. Our business effectively came to a halt in the middle of what was, to date, the busiest March of our career."

A recession is, in its own way, a contagion. From closed shops and beleaguered companies, the disease spreads, triggering mass job loss, missed bills, evictions. The economic consequences of the COVID-19 lockdown cascaded through many industries that heavily employ women: hospitality, service, retail, recreation, arts and entertainment, but also, perhaps surprisingly, health care and social services—making it the first recession in Canadian history that is service-driven. All told, the pandemic plummeted women's participation in the labour force to 55 per cent, its lowest point in three decades. In the first two months alone, 1.5 million women lost their jobs, sparking the term "she-cession." Women in the core working ages, between twenty-five and fifty-four, lost more than twice the number of jobs lost by men in the same age range. But if women's losses were unprecedented, so too was their ability to fix it. "On both sides—on both the carnage as well as the pick-up-the-pieces side—women are for the first time leading economic responses through public policies and through market actions," Armine Yalnizyan, an economist and Atkinson Fellow on the Future of Workers, told CBC's *The*

Current in March. Meaning, women were driving the losses, but they were also, in many cases, driving the recovery.

Women could be forgiven, however, if it felt like they only saw evidence of the carnage. Before CERB was announced on March 25, and before the program began accepting applications on April 6, tens of thousands of Canadians who had already lost their jobs overloaded the country's antiquated EI system. On one early Monday in March, people filed 71,000 claims, punching through the previous single-day record of 38,000 set during the 2008 recession. They broke the record again just a few days later, filing 87,000 claims. By the end of March, the government had 2.2 million EI claims on its virtual desk. People waited for hours and, more often, days to get through to Service Canada's information line. One man reported making 1,700 phone calls before he got through, while others enlisted friends' and partners' phones to call from multiple numbers at once. To help with the overload, and in anticipation that CERB would trigger an avalanche on Employment and Social Development Canada, the government quickly recruited 1,500 volunteers from within to work the phone lines. In the end, about 7,000 people raised their hands to step outside their regular jobs and help answer calls. And still call times stretched like Guinness World taffy. Many people reported calling dozens of times before getting through, only to gratefully make it to the next step: listening to elevator music for, very possibly, their entire day. Or, as one woman put it in mid-April, "Finally got put on hold for three hours . . . made two loaves of banana bread and at 4:35 p.m. they answered. I swear I cried."

By the end of September, at the program's close, more than 8.8 million people had accessed CERB, totalling $80.62 billion in government relief. Many of them had stayed on CERB for months, holding tight to the lifeline. For plenty of women, and particularly mothers, the line frayed anyway—even if it didn't snap. One twenty-seven-year-old single mother from Ontario who lost her job at the beginning of the pandemic shared that she was no longer able to afford medication for her rheumatoid arthritis. After taking care of rent, covering utilities, and paying for her baby's needs, she had only $200 left every month to buy gas and food. She was forced to skip bills, and felt the pain settle in joints. "My baby has everything he needs and that's what you got to do," she said in May. "I'll live on pasta as long as I have to." Another mom, who lives in B.C. with her boyfriend and two children, said that, while CERB ensured the family's survival, it was barely enough; under the program, and while keeping one of her jobs as a part-time server, she still brought in anywhere from $1,300 to $2,300 less each month. CERB didn't quite cover her rent. Without her partner's help, she would have been in a "scary situation": unable to buy food or pay her bills. "Sadly," she acknowledged, "I'm not the only one."

In many ways, CERB helped to normalize social assistance. In the process, it squashed—or, at the very least, stepped on— stigmas about who needed to access such programs, and why.

People who once uttered, "I would never . . ." and "Only lazy people . . ." found themselves without jobs, without opportunities, and yet with plenty of bills and basic needs. More revolutionary, however, were all the renewed conversations about, and demands for, a universal basic income (UBI). The unforeseen and ultra-accelerated economic quake, and with it the introduction of CERB, underscored the precarity of many Canadians. People who'd never heard of a UBI, or had perhaps dismissed its need, were newly open to the conversation. Suddenly, a program under which everyone is guaranteed basic earnings didn't seem so far-fetched. Advocates pushed for Trudeau to pledge its implementation in his September throne speech, and for a while it felt like he would. He didn't (quite), but all the speculation only forced UBI more into the mainstream conversation, something that was, largely, previously unthinkable. "COVID brought us face to face with the fact that stuff happens that is beyond anybody's control," said Dana Wylie, who organized a basic-income rally in September in Edmonton. Before the virus, she hadn't been involved at all in the issue; the pandemic changed her mind. "Yes, the government stepped up and helped but what that made me realize is that this happens to families all the time."

But, for all its positives, CERB wasn't a panacea. The temporary relief could do little to address the flip side of the "she-cession"; that is, the need for a so-called "she-covery." As the economy haltingly—and in some cases, seemingly rapidly—reopened, many women were left behind. They did not recover their jobs at the same rate as men, and for multiple reasons. Fields that tend to employ more women, like the hospitality industry and administrative services companies, face significantly longer recovery periods, at eight and five years respectively. Compare that to construction or manu-facturing, which, by fall 2020, were looking at significantly shorter recovery timelines of just over one year. And reduced child care services added another set of house-sized concrete hurdles to women's back-to-work paths. As one woman said in May, "Do I find a job first? Do I find child care? How do I do one without the other?" Between February and May, employ-ment among parents with toddlers or school-aged kids fell more for mothers than fathers, and more still for single moth-ers. One report found that, while women accounted for about 45 per cent of the decline in hours during the initial downturn, they would only make up 35 per cent of the recovery.

At the same time, the economic infusion—for some—also prompted the government to discontinue CERB in October, precipitating plenty of panic, even as promises of a smooth transition back to an expanded EI program abounded. "I feel almost caged," said one mother in Winnipeg who was still unable to return to work. "I've been put in some type of situa-tion where I have to sit there and deal with whatever comes my way, and I have no control over it." Many women were left wondering how they'd pay back any CERB payments they received in error—a not uncommon mistake made by the gov-ernment in the rush to provide assistance. Others wondered how they'd later pay the required income taxes that came with CERB. Almost all wondered what they could possibly do next. Every day seemed to bring on a new anxiety, their grip on the lifeline feeling a little looser. To make matters worse, the end to eviction bans had a parallel timeline. Already in April, Ontario landlords, for example, had reported a 10 per cent delinquency rate, a tenfold increase from the usual 1 per cent. At that time, one tenants' advocate predicted a "bloodbath" when the ban officially ended, and for many people that was now coming true. And around the same time, about 760,000 Canadians had deferred mortgage payments coming due. "It's a limit that you thought you'd never have to hit," said the Winnipeg mom, speaking of the resulting stress. "And then you hit it. And you have to hit it again the next day." That's to say nothing at all of the women who couldn't access CERB—or any other form of government assistance—in the first place.

On paper, twenty-five-year-old Maryama Ahmed had done everything right. The political science major graduated from the University of Toronto in fall 2019, becoming the first person in her immediate family to earn a bachelor's degree. Photos from that day show Ahmed cradling a bouquet of apricot roses, her gaze focused on something in the distance—possibly her future. And by all accounts, her future did look good. Over the next few months Ahmed applied for, and got accepted into, graduate school at Memorial University of

Newfoundland to further her study in political science. In the meantime, she decided to get a full-time job to pay off her student loans, save for school, and support herself. In February 2020, she was hired for a front-desk position at a downtown Toronto hotel, not too far from her apartment. Her first day was in early March, and Ahmed was excited: her colleagues seemed great, the job paid well, and she had full-time benefits. She was also proud of herself. After growing up in a low-income household, and working a bevy of part-time and contract jobs throughout school, she had found security. A third feeling mixed in: safety. If the path to successful, stable adulthood came with a to-do list, she was checking off every box.

But in the first week of her new job, warning signs already dotted the hotel. After some early scares, the hotel had put a quarantine process in place. Hand sanitizer stations decorated the lobby, halls, every floor. Ahmed remembered thinking that, outside of a hospital, she'd never seen so many installed in one place. The safety measures she'd learned in training had already changed—become more intense, more detailed, more extensive. Within a few days, employees had their hours slashed. "Honestly," Ahmed told her fellow trainees, "we shouldn't be surprised if we get laid off." She just didn't think it would happen so quickly. On March 18, an email from work detonated her inbox, announcing, "Unfortunately, we are shutting down operations." The email listed a tentative reopening date, but Ahmed had a feeling the pandemic would follow an old adage. That is, things in the city would get significantly worse before they got better. She predicted the hotel wouldn't reopen when it planned, and it didn't. The date kept getting pushed back. Ahmed had bills and rent to pay, food to buy, thirty thousand dollars in student debt, and now no income. She watched every update from Prime Minister Trudeau, following every scrap of news, waiting for a relief program. "When the government announced CERB, I thought, 'Oh wow,'" she said, "'This is going to be for me. I lost my job because of COVID-19.'"

Except, it wasn't. To be eligible for CERB, an applicant had to have earned at least five thousand dollars in the previous twelve months. Ahmed hadn't been at her job long enough to meet the threshold. She'd worked a bit over the summer, and had done some tutoring throughout the school year, but it all put her just shy of five thousand dollars, an amount that felt arbitrary to her. Ahmed was dismayed, but she knew the government was also introducing the Canada Emergency Student Benefit, and so held out hope. That would be where she'd fit. But it excluded her, too. Only those who had finished in December 2019 or later were eligible. It included students who were starting in the fall, but not graduate students, like her. She also hadn't accumulated enough hours to qualify for EI. She felt like she was being punished for graduating too early and finding a job too late. She had always done what everyone tells young adults to do if they want a happy, prosperous life, and somehow it still hadn't worked out. "I went to post-secondary. I got the degree. I've never gotten into any trouble," she said. "And so, here I was a productive member of society. I had gotten the job. I was ready to work the forty hours on that job. Then I lost that job because of circumstances that were completely out of my hands—circumstances that nobody saw coming." And nothing existed to catch her.

Ahmed went into survival mode. It's a place, she noted, that she's been in before. Her parents immigrated to Canada from Somalia, and Ahmed grew up in subsidized housing in the Kitchener, Ontario, area. As she put it, "You don't have the luxury to not think about money. It's always in the back of your mind." Once she moved to Toronto for school, she'd always been adamant about ensuring she could sustain herself. To her, the pandemic felt like old worry: worry about paying her bills, worry about paying rent, worry about spending money on any necessity, worry about spending money on something that she didn't really need, worry about spending any money at all. Sometimes, she felt angry and frustrated. She'd done everything right, followed all the advice, and it still felt like she had done nothing right. To make it through, she had to dip into her savings—money that she'd planned to use to pay off her student debt. She had to remind herself that it wasn't her fault; she'd done her due diligence. Her friends and family helped. She used them as a support system whenever she needed to vent. To help keep her mental health intact, she also turned to advocacy organizations, joining Don't Forget Students. The national campaign has worked to bring awareness to people who were in a similar, if not the exact same, boat as Ahmed. It gave her a sense of connection, eased the gnawing sense of helplessness.

In early August, Ahmed shared her story on the organization's Twitter account. She wasn't quite sure what to expect. Ahmed is a self-described open, talkative person, but she rarely used Twitter. She wanted to be honest, and she was. It was the first time she truly took in the difficulty, and trauma, of the previous few months—really, of the past few years; trying to make it through school in Toronto had put her into survival mode, too, more than once. She hadn't shared the full extent of her hustle with her friends and family, hadn't shared all the times she struggled to eat, hadn't told anybody how close to the line she lived in Toronto, what it took to keep up. Doing so now made her feel exposed. But she wanted people to know how bad it could be; she wanted to make a difference. "I don't come from Bill Morneau's world," she wrote, referencing her local member of Parliament (who, incidentally, she said she'd reached out to earlier for help, with no response). "I'm a Black, Muslim woman, born to first-generation immigrants." She continued: "It's been six months since the beginning of Canada's emergency response to COVID-19. I still haven't received any financial support from the federal government." The reaction to her Twitter thread was immediate and overwhelming. People were outraged. Hundreds of them retweeted the post. Many of them called on their own MPs to help.

The experience helped reiterate what motivated her to pursue politics in the first place: every person's responsibility to fight against injustice. Her own experiences as a Black, Muslim woman had shown her that people can face the grind of injustice every day. At the same time, many feasible, non-radical solutions—like universal basic income—existed and could, arguably, be easily implemented. Those solutions could help so many people. "So, there's no excuses, right?" said Ahmed. When we spoke, she told me that she wasn't sure what her dream job would be. She wanted to try a few things: working in government, working for a non-profit, and, sure, one day running for office. She shared that, after Morneau resigned later that month amid the WE Charity controversy, one of her friends held an intervention. "Look," he told her. "You have to run for Morneau's seat." He wouldn't leave her alone about it. "I'm serious," he said. "You've got to do it." She told him, not yet. She was still figuring things out. But the idea of one day shaking up the status quo? Of doing leadership differently? Of setting a tone of compassion and action, not cynicism and apathy? Well, yes, that all sounded like a future she wanted.

"I THINK IT'S IMPORTANT TO CRY. SO MUCH SUFFERING HAS HAPPENED."

Dr. Deena Hinshaw,
Alberta's chief medical officer of health

Seven

EVERY DECISION COUNTS

Deena Hinshaw's daily press conferences could reasonably be renamed Guided Meditation for Pandemic Times. When the provincial chief medical officer of health takes the podium, her voice is calm, clear, and steady—her competence and directness combine to feel grounding, not unlike gently spattering rain, softly trilling birds, or your own deep breaths. This effect remains in place even, and perhaps especially, when she delivers the details of Alberta's sobering new reality. "Previously shared yesterday, as you know, I was tested for COVID-19," opened Hinshaw, in an address to the province on March 17, 2020, St. Patrick's Day. "And I am pleased to let you know that my test results were negative and that I am feeling better this morning." She went on to order the province's first set of public health measures: a limit on mass gatherings and a closure of everything from casinos and bingo halls to libraries and swimming pools to bars and nightclubs. "I know this will disappoint many," she acknowledged, "but we must take action." She continued with why the restrictions were important, and how they would help the entire province. She explained the concept of flattening the curve. And again and again she refused to minimize how much it all would suck. "The measures introduced today will be hard on all of us," she closed, "but I believe we are ready and able to rise to the challenge before us."

During the briefing, Hinshaw wore a grey dress, with the periodic table emblazoned across her arms and chest. The very cool, very scientific wardrobe choice seemed to further win over anxious Albertans. Within days, media had declared, "Alberta Loves Dr. Hinshaw, and Her Periodic Table Dress." It was a fair assumption. Tweets praising the doctor flooded social media. "Can we take a moment to recognize how cool Dr. Hinshaw is?" wrote one user, gushing over both dress and doctor. "How is she not Alberta's premier?" Another Albertan wrote, "Is it too soon to talk about the fact that Dr. Hinshaw has the periodic table on her dress and that I want to be her when I grow up?" Some fans joked that she could have a share of their hoarded toilet paper, while others noted that if Hinshaw could come to their "collective houses and read Albertans a bedtime story we'd all be sleeping better." An Edmonton singer-songwriter crafted lyrics that included the lines, "She's saving all the octogenarians / She reminds me of one of my favourite librarians." And, after being pleasantly bombarded with requests for the dress—and praise for Hinshaw—the garment's B.C.-based designer decided to re-release the previously discontinued design. It sold out almost immediately. The description for the dress now notes, "Yes, this is the dress you've been seeing Dr. Deena Hinshaw wearing on the news."

The dress was only the beginning. In the early months of the pandemic, Hinshaw was ushered into the role of province-wide folk hero—whether she wanted the newfound fame or not (she didn't). Fuelling all that adoration, however, was one difficult decision after another. At the same press conference where she wore The Dress, a journalist asked Hinshaw to clarify whether the new public health rules were based on her recommendations. They were, of course. Though she had an excellent team, and the combined knowledge of the other provincial and territorial health officers across the country, the weight of the province's health decisions ultimately teetered on her shoulders. It was "absolutely unnerving," said Hinshaw, to rely on the rapidly evolving, question-inducing information about the virus to make those decisions. She didn't have a crystal ball, she couldn't see into the future; she had to make decisions based on what she knew, and nobody knew very much at all.

What they did know could easily fast-forward out of date. In one Friday briefing in March, she swore that she would not close schools. On Monday, she closed them. Hinshaw had to make a lot of one-eighty decisions like that: telling people asymptomatic carriers couldn't transmit the virus, then warning they could; saying don't wear masks, then definitely do. If the virus was a monster, it was a shapeshifting one. Blink once and it looked like influenza. Blink again and it looked like

SARS. Blink a third time and it looked like neither of those things. Alberta didn't get its first case until March 5—so much later than the other provinces that Hinshaw actually wondered if the new coronavirus had arrived in Alberta undetected. She felt the same awful anticipation so many others have described. She wondered, briefly, if something about Alberta was protecting the province. Then everything moved in a hundred directions, thousands of rubber bands snapping. All the theoretical plans already in place were considered and, one by one, gradually abandoned. "In the time span between when we had our first case and two weeks later," Hinshaw said, "we did many things that were beyond what we had originally anticipated." From that point on, it was a blur.

The SARS-CoV-2 virus is unthinking and unfeeling. It goes without saying that the virus doesn't have a gender equality agenda. Nonetheless, it has managed to upend every historical and cultural reference we have for who should lead us through crisis, and how. Across Canada, and in countries around the world, compassion, kindness, and collaboration rose like cream throughout the first year of the pandemic—largely thanks to the women leaders who embraced these traits. We gravitated toward people like Hinshaw, B.C.'s Bonnie Henry, the federal government's Theresa Tam, and P.E.I.'s Heather Morrison precisely because they seemed to eschew the bravado, brashness, and unwavering ego that makes many male leaders so

popular, in both the present and past. These women were neither certain nor infallible; they were honest and human. It
made them all the more compelling, all the more comforting.
Arguably, their fanbase grew not because they were untouch-
able or because they gave rousing, ear-blistering speeches, but
because they communicated clearly, consistently, and with
others' best interests at heart. Their lives felt attainable. They
struggled just like you, broke just like you, knew it was hard
and impossible, just like you. If this vulnerability and relatabil-
ity felt surprising, it also felt necessary.

Alison Van Rosendaal, an assistant principal in Calgary, said
of Hinshaw, "I just love watching her." Van Rosendaal believes
that media, government, and plain general discourse have con-
ditioned many of us to expect populist rhetoric and, in return,
to fit our own response to any issue, no matter how complex,
into equally rigid camps. She appreciated that Hinshaw didn't
turn all the crowded fear into a blunt instrument, that she
seemed uninterested in both soundbites and easy solutions.
"She let the things that were messy, stay messy," said Van
Rosendaal, explaining what drew her to the unofficial Hinshaw
fan club. "She repeatedly said, 'We don't have the solution. We
don't have the knowledge base. We don't have the research.'"
Rather than that feeling frustrating, however—as in, "Well
what *do* you have?"—it felt refreshing. Van Rosendaal had
only to look at the U.S. to see what could happen when political agendas infiltrated infectious disease management, how

false claims and disingenuous solutions could ransack a country's response. Hinshaw might have to apologize for getting public policy wrong every now and then, but at least nobody was drinking bleach.

Van Rosendaal remembered the March 16 briefing, before Hinshaw announced her (first) negative COVID-19 test, as the one that won her over. That day, Hinshaw had addressed the province from home, via a flat screen, seated in front of walls lined with book shelves. She talked about how she was isolating herself from her family and about the configuration of her house, acknowledging how tough it was and recognizing her privilege for being able to do so. It struck Van Rosendaal, who has three children, including one teenager, and also three grandchildren, that Hinshaw was doing a difficult, demanding job within the same constraints she'd asked everyone else to work within—and that she wasn't afraid to admit it. At the time, Van Rosendaal was watching the briefing across the street at her sister's house (though within two weeks, she and her sister would be staying isolated in their own homes). The two joked that they needed Hinshaw T-shirts. As they talked about how much they appreciated Hinshaw and batted around ideas on what, exactly, those shirts would look like, and what a tagline might be, a lightbulb clicked on for Van Rosendaal: "What Would Dr. Hinshaw Do?"

Her sister loved it, and Van Rosendaal decided she'd actually get one made, solely because it would be amusing. They'd laugh, and have a fun shirt to wear with their new hero on it.

Shortly after, she was awake in bed at 2:30 a.m. on a Wednesday, staring at her ceiling, thinking about the shirt. Unable to sleep, Van Rosendaal went to her computer and transformed a screenshot photo of Hinshaw with her hands open wide. She gave her sunglasses and a rope of necklaces, centring the cheeky, and not-quite-rhetorical, question on the black-and-white rendering. She got ten shirts made, keeping one for herself and giving the others to her sister, as well as to some local health heroes. Her delighted sister, Julie, a cookbook author and food editor, posted a photo of the shirt on her social media accounts, where her followers all immediately seemed to want one. One person posted, "I am very, very, very jealous right now." Others suggested the design should go on an infinity scarf (another favourite Hinshaw fashion choice) or should come with a periodic table print. One comment in particular seemed to sum it all up: "I know everyone's asking, but are these for sale?"

"It was this common sentiment bubbling up of, 'Oh, we love her,'" Van Rosendaal told me. She found a small manufacturer in nearby Red Deer and decided to make a few shirts, sell them, and give the proceeds to some local food banks. She picked ten organizations across Alberta, including several located in Indigenous communities. It would be easy enough, she thought, to do this one good thing. In fact, she was volunteering at a 5 p.m. shift at a food bank shortly after announcing the shirt sale when her phone started chiming notifications. Safety precautions meant she couldn't touch her phone during the shift, so Van Rosendaal had to listen and wonder. *Ching, ching, ching.* By the end of the shift, she'd already sold two thousand dollars' worth of shirts. The next day, sales had climbed so high she thought, *This is no longer a lark* and *Shit, I should have asked Dr. Hinshaw if this was okay.* She reached out, and Hinshaw gave an uncomfortable blessing. Within four days, Van Rosendaal had sold more than twenty thousand dollars in T-shirts. She can't be sure why the shirts were so popular, but she thinks it was because, to many people, Hinshaw felt like hope.

"These new heroes that are coming out of the pandemic are such a positive for the world," said Mandy Stobo, "not just for the pandemic, but forever." Stobo is a Calgary-based artist who is known for her Bad Portrait series—bright pop-art watercolour-and-Sharpie portraits of people she admires. She created one of Hinshaw first, inspired by the doctor's bravery, determination, and poise. Soon after, Stobo started creating portraits of other healthcare workers and health officers. "Once you look past Alberta," she added, "it was pretty consistent: the theme of these incredible women taking the pandemic by the horns and steering us in the right direction." She created colourful portraits of Henry and Tam, then added Newfoundland's Janice Fitzgerald, Ottawa's Vera Etches, and Toronto's Eileen de Villa. To her, each woman had become a modern icon worth lauding. Stobo decided to license the portraits for free to people who were doing fundraisers, helping however she could. In doing so, she joined Van Rosendaal and countless others who had decided to publicly honour Canada's new set of leaders with T-shirts, art, shoes, fundraisers, songs, graffiti, fan clubs, signs, coffee mugs, stationery, and more. The accolades vibrated against the fear, an undercurrent of appreciation, admiration, and support.

It isn't often we see women leaders so widely celebrated during a crisis—in part because it's still far too uncommon for us to see women lead communities and countries at all (not to mention companies, courtrooms, civil organizations, media rooms, and the list goes on). The reversal did not go unnoticed in Canada and beyond. In addition to Tam's chief spot at the federal level, six of the top doctors in the country's thirteen provinces and territories were women. So too were many health officers at the municipal level. Together, they showed us a new way to lead. They defied hate, deliberate misinformation, partisanship. Tam openly, repeatedly condemned anti-Asian racism. (Whereas some male leaders, such as Ontario Conservative MP David Sloan, who asked "Does [Tam] work for China?" and tweeted "Dr. Tam must go! Canada must remain sovereign over decisions," instead focused on sowing division.) Henry's signature phrase, "Be kind, be calm, be safe," became the country's unofficial mantra. We connected so deeply to these women of the pandemic not because they were perfect or unhindered, but because, in so many ways, they were us: frazzled and afraid, determined and compassionate, facing down an unfathomable future, each of them simply doing the best that they could. Under pressure, these women were graceful and stoic, but also tired, sad, and keenly aware of loss.

Their voices broke when they talked about missing their families. They choked back tears when they acknowledged just how hard it all was, and asked us to keep doing everything that made it hard. "I ended up showing some emotion in public—not because I wanted to, but because it happened. It made it real for all of us," Heather Morrison, P.E.I.'s chief health officer, told me, referring to a press conference during which she asked Islanders to continue being patient, to continue being kind. "I wouldn't recommend crying on TV, but it happened." The honesty only made people love her more. An MLA named a new calf after her. Kids hosted a virtual superhero-themed party and some dressed up as her. Like with other leaders, people made T-shirts with her likeness on them—a thing that Morrison said she would never have believed, not in a million years, if you'd told her at the beginning of 2020. She has tried her best to be a calm voice in the storm. Similar to Hinshaw, she has not shied away from admitting errors and has been upfront about what she does, and does not, know. She too led with compassion, kindness, patience, and common sense. She too put everyone else—her entire province—first.

This near-universal approach from women leaders wasn't just humane; it was effective. When I spoke to Morrison in early August, for example, her tiny province had experienced no COVID-19 deaths; that remained the case into October.

At the international level, studies of the world's 194 countries have shown that women national leaders fared better in terms of both infection and mortality rates. One possible reason, researchers found, is that, unlike men, women appeared to approach the crisis with one top mandate: to save lives. On average, they announced lockdowns twenty-five deaths earlier than their male counterparts. For better or worse, during the first wave, they prioritized health over the economy. These leaders totalled fewer than twenty and notably included Germany's Angela Merkel, New Zealand's Jacinda Ardern, Denmark's Mette Frederiksen, Taiwan's Tsai Ing-wen, and Finland's Sanna Marin. (To account for the disparity in numbers, the study compared each woman-led country with an analogous, nearby male-led one.)

As the *Guardian* put it, "Plenty of countries with male leaders . . . have done well. But few with female leaders have done badly." In April, the *Atlantic* even posited that Ardern might be "the most effective leader on the planet" for the way she was handling the pandemic. In the early months, she exemplified empathy but also an unbreakable commitment to valuing human life before anything else. As Ardern herself said when she announced increased mass shutdowns in her country, "The worst-case scenario is simply intolerable. It would represent the greatest loss of New Zealanders' lives in our country's history. I will not take that chance." And neither would many others.

———

Kami Kandola wasn't about to wait for the Northwest Territories to get its first case. On March 18, in response to her urging, the territory declared a public health emergency—an order it would go on to extend at least fourteen times. As the N.W.T.'s chief public health officer, and someone who had been working in the North for more than seventeen years, Kandola knew the vast expanse of land wasn't particularly populous. In fact, at just under forty-five thousand people, the entire territory was smaller than most suburban cities in Canada. Some of the N.W.T.'s thirty-three communities are home to only about a hundred people; one, Kakisa, has fewer than fifty residents. Many of them are only accessible by plane, and few of them are linked to major roads. In some ways, their remoteness made them seem like the safest places in Canada to avoid community transmission. Certainly, that's why in March 2020 one misguided Quebec couple sold their possessions and attempted to flee to Old Crow, an Indigneous community of 250, located in Yukon, one territory over from the N.W.T. The community's chief, Dana Tizya-Tramm, politely told them to get lost. Old Crow could barely house the residents it did have; there was no space for the couple. More than that, though, he had the same fear as Kandola: that one COVID-19 case could raze a far-flung Indigenous community in the North. Their protection was in their isolation; break it and, potentially, break everything.

"I know how outbreaks can be started," said Kandola. "When it comes to infectious diseases Indigenous communities bear the brunt of the burden." That has been true for more than three hundred years, starting when settlers first brought tuberculosis (TB) to the southeast. By the 1930s and '40s, the TB death rate among those living on reserves was the highest ever reported in a human population. The next decade, at least one-third of Inuit were infected. By 2008, the TB rate among Indigenous people was six times higher than the overall Canadian rate. In Nunavut, it was thirty-eight times the national average. And while tuberculosis provides one of the starkest examples, it's well documented that Indigenous peoples across Canada experience higher rates of heart disease; certain sexually transmitted infections, including HIV/AIDS; some cancers; and even dementia. Rates of diabetes are staggeringly higher—a particular concern during the COVID-19 outbreak, as the disease has been reported to drastically elevate risk of serious damage from the virus.

For a recent example of the unique vulnerabilities of Indigenous communities, Kandola and others tasked with protecting such populations could also turn to the 2009 H1N1 pandemic. Those living in First Nation communities were 2.8 times more likely to be hospitalized from the flu strain, and had an ICU admission rate that was three times higher than that of non-Indigenous people. Or, put another way: while Indigenous people represent only 4.3 per cent of the population, during the first wave of H1N1 they accounted for 27.8 per cent of hospitalizations and made up 25.6 per cent of critically ill patients in ICUs across Canada. A history of colonialism and the resulting and persistent inequities, together with the very isolation that could potentially protect communities from SARS-CoV-2, hold much of the blame for such poor health outcomes—both directly and indirectly. Colonial policies and legislation in Canada are, as many Indigenous rights advocates have said, a pandemic unto themselves. For centuries, this complex web has perpetuated countless socio-economic, cultural, and political injustices, many of which, in turn, make it hard to fend off an unyielding killer virus.

Chronic disease is a risk factor. Crowded, multi-generational housing is a risk factor. Poverty is a risk factor. Dirty water is a risk factor. Poor nutrition is a risk factor. Lack of access to dependable health care is a risk factor. Discriminatory and racist health care is a risk factor. Low trust is a risk factor. Delayed and badly communicated public health information is a risk factor. A history of low and no resources is a risk factor. The remoteness that made the region seem so attractive to naive southerners is a risk factor. As Kandola herself acknowledged, most communities in the North don't have easy access to a hospital. A number of them don't even have a permanent nurse on site every day. Treatment would be slow, if it came at all. "If we get the novel coronavirus in our communities," Kandola asserted, "it will spread." Unless, of course, she acted quickly and decisively.

The N.W.T. confirmed its first case of COVID-19 on March 21, hours before closing its borders to non-essential visitors. Kandola told me she'd already made the decision to shut the territory to air, road, and port travel before a resident in Yellowknife tested positive. She had been watching the case counts climb in the provinces to the immediate south and wanted to be proactive. She wanted to make wise use of the time she had before the virus arrived—even if, as it turned out, she didn't have any time at all. By that point, the territory had already administered hundreds of COVID-19 tests, and it planned to keep administering them aggressively, despite the low case count. The first positive test belonged to a person who'd travelled to Alberta and B.C. before returning home, just as Kandola anticipated might happen. The person and their family were told to self-isolate after receiving the diagnosis and did so, immediately. Then, Kandola and her team tracked down seventy people who had come into contact with that person and prescribed another round of mandatory isolation. Over the next few weeks, another four people tested positive in the territory. The last of them recovered without incident in mid-April, and nobody else tested positive for months.

Throughout it all, Kandola remained vigilant. She worked constantly, through evenings and weekends, describing the period as "intense." The idea of 5 p.m. signalling the day's end became laughable; seeing her family, a husband and four children, became near impossible. In a way, it was almost familiar, too: during H1N1, Kandola had missed her youngest son's first birthday; she's missed a lot of stuff this time around, as well. During the non-stop early days, an epidemiologist on her team presented Kandola with a superhero cape, calling her "Super Kami." She hung it on the back of her chair, thinking of all the *Avengers* movies she'd been watching with her twelve-year-old son. "It's a flavour of how our team is dealing with the pandemic. The mentality is that it's not just about you—you are trying to protect society at large and the people you love and care about need you to be focused," she said. "They need you to put their needs before yours." She took the philosophy to heart as she led her morning huddles, and, as she began making tough decisions to protect her real-life population, she hoped everyone else would too.

At her order, restaurants, gyms, schools, and some offices remained closed until the territory ticked into June. At the end of August, a checkpoint in Hay River, close to the Alberta border, was still refusing entry to at least a dozen vehicles a day. As fall hit, the territory enacted mandatory mask measures at airports, and so too did many stores. By October 9, the N.W.T. had completed over 5,570 virus tests, and the number of COVID-positive results never budged. Nor did Kandola, even as criticism of too-strict measures surfaced in the territory, as it did elsewhere in Canada. Much of that grumbling arrived as she and her team prepared for what Kandola saw as the inevitable second wave—there hadn't yet been a pandemic in history without one. And indeed, after a months-long virus drought, the N.W.T. recorded three new cases in mid-October. Kandola knew they were coming. For her, the previous six months had only been a drill; the real test was still on its way.

Standing at the base of another possible mountain, she vowed to put even stricter precautions in place if she had to. After all, she said, examples of worst-case scenarios abounded. In particular, she looked with worry to northern Saskatchewan, a public health failure close to home—and a place similar in both population size and demographics to the N.W.T. "You can never know how much prevention stopped," she said, "but we know by looking at unmitigated public health measures what *could* have happened."

On April 15, Saskatchewan's far north reported its first COVID-19 case in La Loche, a Dene village that's home to about 2,800 people. Health officials later confirmed that the virus's arrival in the community was linked to travel from an oil sands camp in Alberta. The virus quickly spread. By the time the province restricted non-critical travel to the province's north eleven days later, the area accounted for twenty-five of the fifty-seven active cases. The communities dotted there faced the same challenges as those in the N.W.T., and, arguably, in every Indigenous community and reserve across Canada. When housing is overcrowded and inadequate, self-isolation doesn't work no matter how hard people try, or how responsible they are. The virus pillaged the region for three months. By the time the last active case was deemed recovered in July, the area accounted for nearly one-third of COVID-19 infections in Saskatchewan. More than two hundred people in La Loche got sick, and another sixty-two became ill in nearby Clearwater River Dene Nation. Some died.

And it wasn't, of course, simply Indigenous people in remote areas who faced higher risks.

"I mean, the system is racist everywhere," said Lisa Richardson, an Indigenous internist at Toronto General Hospital. "There is so much systemic racism. There is individual racism. There is structural racism, and there is epistemic racism." Richardson is also the vice-chair of culture and inclusion at University of Toronto's School of Medicine and the lead strategic advisor in Indigenous health for both U of T's Faculty of Medicine and Women's College Hospital. Richardson has thought a lot about what it means to offer trauma-informed, anti-racist, culturally safe care in the time of COVID-19. She knows that many Indigenous people mistrust the healthcare system and the privilege-steeped idea that it is there to help them feel better, to keep their bodies and their minds healthy—and for good reason. Even when they do enter the system, Richardson added, they face major barriers to treatment, including a dearth of humane and culturally safe care. That might mean, for example, a doctor who doesn't understand they are treating a patient who's been to residential school and been forced to undergo medical procedures. Or it might mean hospital staff who are blatantly racist and cruel, callously endangering their patients' lives.

Consider the tragic, deplorable death of Joyce Echaquan. The thirty-seven-year-old Atikamekw woman and mother of seven drove three hours from her home in Manawan to a hospital in Joliette, Quebec, one Saturday morning in late

September 2020. Echaquan sought help for her severe stomach pain and also suffered from a chronic heart condition. By Monday morning, she was in even worse pain. She feared she was being given morphine, which she was allergic to, and worried she was over-medicated. Nurses only derided her. So, Echaquan began live-streaming her experience on Facebook. It lasted seven minutes, and in it a nurse can be heard saying, in French, "Are you done acting stupid? Are you done?" Echaquan groans in pain, and another nurse joins in. "You made some bad choices, my dear. What are your children going to think, seeing you like this?" The first nurse responds, "She's good at having sex, more than anything else." Her cousin saw the video and, shocked and worried, sped down to the hospital to pick up Echaquan, to get her out of that place. When she arrived, nobody would let her see her cousin or give her any information. Finally, upon discovering why she was there, a nurse told her, "Oh, you don't know yet? She's died."

Indigenous people know all too well that, despite politicians' protestations otherwise, such incidents are far from rare. So, then, how do you convince communities and individuals that public health measures are trying to keep them safe? How do you convince them that getting tested for COVID-19 is a smart idea? Throughout the pandemic, Richardson worked with Anishnawbe Health Toronto's mobile testing unit to try and do exactly that. The mobile unit was designed to bypass the assessment centre and meet Indigenous people where they were at, literally. It travelled to the city's shelters and homeless encampments, but also outside the downtown core, where pockets of Indigenous people live but don't have access to care. Once people agreed to be tested, Richardson practised clear and kind communication, explaining what she was doing and why. If a patient was still, understandably, apprehensive, she learned to offer to let them do the invasive-feeling test themselves. She'd clasp their hand and, thus joined, help guide the swab inside the nose. If that didn't work, she'd offer a throat swab, always taking her cue from the patient. She cites the mobile unit as one example of Indigenous-led health solutions during the pandemic. But there also were many others.

Plenty of communities did shut their borders, and fast. One Inuit association made their own educational materials to disseminate, written in Inuktitut and using common examples from the daily lives of community members. Richardson helped Women's College Hospital adopt a medicine wheel framework that incorporated elder knowledge and focused on building physical, emotional, mental, and spiritual resilience. Through these measures, many Indigenous communities reversed their expected fate: poor outcomes similar to H1N1, only magnified by the scale and force of COVID-19. First Nations, Inuit, and Métis communities actually had *lower* rates of COVID-19 in the first six months of the pandemic. Those on reserve had a virus case rate four times lower than the general population, with three times fewer fatalities and a 30 per cent higher recovery rate. And in La Loche, the outbreak finally ended because all levels of government collaborated—prompted in part by a letter from twenty-four Indigenous communities to the province's CMO that read, "We ask you to learn from us, and with us"—and followed a community-crafted response plan. As Richardson put it to me: it's amazing to see the difference power and control can make.

The pandemic thrust many women into vise-like leadership positions. The trial under near impossible pressure wasn't limited to people in visible, political roles. Everywhere, people had to make decisions with devastating costs, often to prevent even worse fallout. Leadership skills were tested and discovered, and sometimes it really did feel like walking through fire. Nadine Abdullah was in the fourth year of her five-year term as the internal medicine program site director at Toronto Western Hospital when the pandemic struck. As the site director, she's responsible for every internal medicine resident at the hospital. That responsibility includes their training, but Abdullah also acts as their role model, their advocate, their support system, their cheerleader—and all of it together helps shape each resident's career. She realized the enormity of that role during a pandemic while seated in Toronto's Royal Alexandra Theatre watching the musical *Come From Away* in early March. She briefly thought, *We probably shouldn't be here*. Then, she thought, *We have to trust in our public health authorities*. And then, in the middle of the show, the frantic phone calls started: from residents; from colleagues; from faculty at U of T, through which the residency program is run. Everyone wanted to know what they should do. The next day, everything changed. Abdullah had never thought she was a strong leader; she was terrified.

She wasn't scared of everything she'd have to do as a mother: grocery shopping, home-schooling, getting medications renewed. She knew how to plan for all of that. What scared her was working on the hospital's Armageddon plan: scenarios for one hundred patients, two hundred patients, three hundred patients. "That's a war," she said. Abdullah suffers from multiple chronic diseases, including one that requires she take Trump's purported cure-all, hydroxychloroquine, and she worried about potential shortages of said medication. As someone who is at higher risk, she knew she likely wouldn't survive the virus. Would she have to engage in care that would put her own life at risk? How would she learn about the disease if she didn't? And how would she teach her residents about it? And, more than anything, how would she keep them safe? Questions tumbled through her mind, and she had trouble sleeping, night after night. What about PPE? Would there be a shortage? Had the hospital made a mistake in requiring only surgical masks be worn, not N95 masks? Would they run out of ventilators? At first, after ample consideration, she told her site lead that she didn't feel comfortable working with COVID-19 patients; her own health put her at too high of a risk. Then, she applied the same person-by-person approach to each resident. She answered every call and text to her cellphone. She had socially distanced meetings. As she privately dealt with her own fears, she heard theirs. "No one was treated equally," she told me. "It was all about what did everybody need for them?"

She never told her residents about her own health problems, or let on that she might be more scared than they were. As April advanced, she decided that she no longer wanted to hide from COVID. If her residents were in a position where they might have to look after virus patients, she had to face it, too—no matter the risk. She wanted to show them she could be their leader; she could be on the COVID-19 team. And that first shift? "It was nothing." She felt safe in her PPE. At home, she quarantined in her basement, taking her dinner to the top of the stairs to eat together with, but apart from, her husband and two children. They'd prop up her phone and watch *Kim's Convenience* together. She began to feel like she was getting a grip on leading through the pandemic.

That new confidence cracked shortly after, in the beginning of May. Around that time, four COVID-19 outbreaks shook Toronto Western, spreading to nineteen patients and forty-six staff members. Hospitals were set to rotate residents, and suddenly none of them wanted to accept anybody who had been working at Toronto Western. Panic set in and a well-intentioned U of T intervened to create its own policies. Unfortunately, the resulting memo failed to properly communicate with hospitals or residents, adding havoc to the mix. On Monday, many residents didn't show up to work, as directed in the memo. Abdullah called a town hall to clarify what had happened, to apologize, and to explain how the hospital and university would move forward together. It didn't go well. Or, as Abdullah said, "It was a disaster."

Emotions ran high. While most residents seemed to understand, several wouldn't accept the explanation and they became aggressive, even vitriolic, she told me. They accused the hospital and program of using residents as human shields. "I can't tell you how I felt I failed," said Abdullah. "I just couldn't control the tears." She did take it personally, and, in her next meeting, offered to resign. Logically, she knew that she hadn't done anything wrong. She knew that she, and everyone else, had made the best decisions they could, given the constraints; other decisions, and mistakes, had been out of her control. At the same time, she also felt like the town hall was a vote of non-confidence; she felt like maybe she wasn't doing a good job after all. But her resignation wasn't accepted. Her colleagues and her own superiors wanted to keep her in leadership. Her own children and her husband told her: we hear you on your daily calls; those residents need you.

When I spoke with her months later, she was still upset and seemed ambivalent about staying in her position. "What people don't understand," she said, "is that we're going through the pandemic, too. We're terrified, too. And we're barely keeping it together." Still, she had kept working with COVID-19 patients, kept helping the residents, and kept wondering if she was doing the right thing, leading the right way, making the best decisions. When it came down to it, like all the new leaders of the pandemic, she had simply kept going, doing it all, even when she wanted to stop.

Hinshaw woke up at 5 a.m. for months. She began her day by working at home before heading to her office. There, she'd read the latest SARS-CoV-2 science and use it to lead decisions on everything from testing strategies to lockdown measures to industry closures. She announced those decisions daily at 3:30 p.m. Back at home, she'd work until 10 or 11 p.m. Then, repeat. Like the virus, Hinshaw's routine was constant and relentless, obliterating breaks, balance, and weekends. Characteristically humble and gracious, she credits her team and her husband, her "greatest cheerleader," for helping her keep it together. Her mother also helped big time, looking after Hinshaw's two elementary school–aged children for half the week at her own house and half the week at her daughter's. Hinshaw's faith tradition grounded her, infusing her with the belief that she is always part of something bigger than herself, one chain-link of connection with the whole. Still, there were days when she didn't feel so Zen. It didn't happen often, but there were times where she had pushed and pushed and pushed for something— or, conversely, had *been* pushed—until she'd finally had enough. She's thankful those rare times happened when she was with supportive people. She could let it out, cry in her office, wipe her eyes, pick herself up, and get back to it. "Honestly," she said, "I think it's important to cry"—to release the grief, to admit despair. "So much suffering has happened—not just as a direct result of the infection, but also the impact on people."

For Hinshaw, the hardest thing is knowing that, despite all the long hours and careful evaluation, she couldn't protect everyone from COVID-19. The second hardest thing is knowing that the same wise decisions she made to protect Albertans rippled out and caused harm: mass unemployment; mass isolation; and, carried on those twin waves like flotsam, a national increase in drug overdoses and substance abuse, in suicide and self-harm, and in domestic violence. Hinshaw became the symbol of both sides of the pandemic—the protective shield and the unintentional wrecking ball. In many other provinces, she said, a few individuals assumed the public face of COVID-19. In Alberta, however, "it's just been me." Consequently, Hinshaw gets a lot of email. Strangers share their deep rage, their concern, their praise, their gratitude, their myriad definitive opinions on what she should do going forward (here, she lets out a sharp, self-deprecating laugh): "Resign." She does read all the feedback, and sifts out everything she finds useful, even when it's critical. In the first month, someone wrote to tell her that, while they appreciated her updates, the daily COVID-19 death toll made it seem like those losses were the only ones that mattered. Since then, Hinshaw has consciously acknowledged that many people are grieving in a time during which grief is especially complicated; she has extended her sympathies to them all. Another person wrote to say that when she was talking about following public safety measures, she only used the word *you*, which felt like a gigantic pointing finger. Hinshaw switched to *we*. She has checked her tone for lecturing, for shaming, for anything that does not suggest we are all in it together.

"I always want to contextualize," Hinshaw told me, "that I'm well aware not every Albertan loves me." Mostly, it doesn't matter. While she appreciates the accolades, she is not on the podium to make herself look good. She is not up there to elevate herself. She stands up there nearly every day simply to share the best information she has, and the best recommendations she can give based on it. If she's wrong, she'll say that too. It's been strange for her to ascend into the public consciousness. When she took the job in January 2019, she knew that she'd have to speak with media. She knew there would be days she would stand at a podium in front of a background of alternating draped maple leaves and folded Rocky Mountains and share important public health information. Like everything else about the scale of the pandemic, though, this magnitude of visibility previously felt impossible. She's had to learn how to express her natural compassion but still build boundaries—to accept she cannot solve everyone's problems. Like other stars, she's also had to learn to keep a part of herself tucked away from the public eye. "I feel like the way I cope with that attention is to recognize that all of that attention is on the Dr. Hinshaw role," she said. "It's almost like, in my own circle, I can then slip out of it and just be me."

The same calm, measured principles she exhibits in press conferences have likewise helped to guide her through the stratosphere. "I've committed to being honest and transparent," she told me, "and to acknowledging when I make mistakes or when something doesn't go well." She thinks that this, more than anything, is what's resonated with Albertans: her ability to concede imperfection. From a lot of people, such sentiments can sound strikingly like a line, a political platitude. And, admittedly, she's said something similar in several other interviews. Coming from Hinshaw, though, it sounds as genuine and down to earth as a Sunday dinner.

For starters, it's true. On May 1, she opened one of her daily briefings with an apology. "In the announcement I made earlier this week regarding visitor restrictions in continuing care, I did not ensure that operators had been fully consulted or notified prior to the policy change," she said. "I am sorry." On the last day in August, she apologized for the confusion her back-to-school updates sparked. And it isn't just that Hinshaw can admit a wrong step. It's that she urges compassion instead of fear, community instead of blame. When she announced a new outbreak of fifty-seven cases at a Calgary-based Ethiopian church, she stressed that members of the church deserved support, not stigma. "An outbreak can occur anywhere," she said, "and those involved need our compassion." That's just the type of leader Hinshaw is. On the day we chatted over video, she was at home. Reaching for a Kleenex, she explained that she had a runny nose and sore throat, so she'd done the responsible thing and self-isolated. She's that kind of leader, too.

"THERE WAS NOT ONE PERSON WHO DIED ALONE. I MADE SURE OF THAT."

Roisin O'Brien,
care aide

Eight

A HIGH TOLL

Death has always been a part of Roisin O'Brien's job. The twenty-seven-year-old had been working at a Vancouver long-term care centre for nearly four years when COVID-19 hit in mid-March. She often sat with people who were in palliative care. She would hold their hand, stroke their hair, make sure they knew she was with them at the end. Many residents didn't have family, either in the city or at all, and O'Brien never wanted them to look around at an empty room. So she'd sit and wait, whether the last breath came in half an hour or an entire shift later. Sometimes it was peaceful, and sometimes it wasn't; no matter what, O'Brien was there. Her job as a care aide is rarely easy. There can be a lot of workplace violence: she's been called names, and right off the top of her head, she can think of at least six times an angry or scared resident has hit her. But this part made it all worth it. O'Brien liked knowing she could spend time with her clients, offer a kind word. She liked knowing that nobody under her care would die alone. She liked knowing that, in that final moment, she did what she could.

As the outbreak ripped through the country, hitting B.C. in late January, O'Brien began to stay home more and more. Her fiancé took over grocery-shopping duties. She didn't want to be the person who brought the virus into her care home. At the same time, she knew that chronic short-staffing often meant people showed up to work sick. Maybe they guiltily dismissed their runny nose as a little sniffle, their sore throat as feeling just a bit scratchy. They didn't want to leave their co-workers hanging. They couldn't afford to pass up the hours. They could manage a shift, they reasoned; they just needed to wear a disposable mask. Before COVID-19, O'Brien had done it, too, figuring that skipping her shift would do more harm. That thinking changed on March 7 when Bonnie Henry announced a COVID-19 outbreak at Lynn Valley Care Centre in North Vancouver, confirming both residents and staff had tested positive. The next night, one of the facility's residents, an eighty-three-year-old man, died, becoming Canada's first COVID-19 death. O'Brien's own care home called a manda-tory staff meeting in response. Sixty people crammed into a 35-square-metre room. They decided to start restricting vis-itors from out of town. They would start asking questions about whether people had recently been abroad. There would be no more coming in sick.

"It turns out, we didn't really have to worry because the virus was already there," said O'Brien. "In hindsight, over half of the people in that room had COVID." Shortly after the meeting, she took an overtime shift on another floor. There was a man there who was vomiting and had diarrhea. O'Brien was worried because she knew his symptoms matched some of the more severe COVID-19 cases. She had no PPE because she hadn't been provided with it, and so she entered his room without any. She breathed the same air and touched her fingertips to his skin. When his condition worsened, she called the ambulance. The paramedics arrived in full virus-armour, "completely gowned up." O'Brien had one scalpel-sharp thought: *What if this is our first case?* The next day, she found out it was. She immediately took her temperature: 38.7 degrees Celsius. A moderate fever. She turned around and headed to a testing clinic. Two days later she got her results and, to her surprise, they were negative. She called her care centre right away and offered to take a shift. In the intervening days, the virus had played hopscotch through the centre. Both residents and facility healthcare workers were sick. She'd work the floor that housed all of the former, she told her supervisors. Hours after offering, she was at work. "And that," she said, "is when all hell broke loose."

Every resident who was sick lived on the dementia floor. Keeping them all quarantined in their rooms was impossible. If they were well enough, they wanted to walk around, they wanted to give O'Brien hugs, they wanted to be close. They touched everything because they didn't understand why they shouldn't. O'Brien would look at empty carts where the PPE was supposed to be and feel a helpless kind of anger boil. She wore the same surgical mask and worked double shift after double shift, from 3 p.m. right on through to 7 a.m. On a normal evening pre-COVID, there would be five care aides, including her, and one nurse. Now they were lucky to have three. Direction from management seemed to change from hour to hour. O'Brien was used to having a list of twelve residents to care for; she could check in several times a night with them, make sure they had everything they needed, stop and chat. Now, in one eight-hour shift, she had to look after forty—changing their adult diapers, sheets, and other incontinence products, washing their bodies and hair, feeding them. She couldn't do it all to the standard she wanted. She didn't have time to wash people's faces. If someone needed changing, she'd do it once, then put them right to bed.

O'Brien had never cried over her job before, but she did now, after every shift and sometimes during them. She'd come home, take a shower, cry, eat, sleep, and then do it all over again. She constantly felt sick to her stomach. Usually, she told me, she tries to distance herself from the tough stuff, summoning the grit to keep going with the mantra *This is my job*. But on the second or third day of working the designated COVID-19 floor, she stopped dissociating, stepped back, and let her brain take a big-picture snapshot of the scene around her. What she saw was horrific. *Oh my god*, she thought. *This is neglect. This isn't right at all.*

By May, the worst-case scenario everyone feared had silently engulfed long-term care facilities across Canada. Cleave them out, and it looked like the country had mainly managed to escape a full-on nightmare during the first wave. There was no broad shortage of PPE inside hospitals. No body bags trimming the hallways. Sirens did not play a soundtrack on the street. Masses of doctors had not been forced into gut-wrenching ethical decisions, choosing who would live and die. Inside care homes, however, a different narrative stretched into chaos. Staff in many facilities reported low or no PPE. In some places, management locked up protective equipment, fearing the staff would steal it, leaving them with nothing to wear on their shifts. New policy and training procedures were developed too slowly, and often, once they were in place, were poorly communicated. Fear and misinformation wormed through countless care centres. Plenty of people quit or got sick, and staffing schedules began to resemble emptied honeycombs. While Canada had a relatively low COVID-19 mortality rate compared to other developed countries, in the initial months of the pandemic it earned the dubious distinction of having the highest proportion of deaths occurring in long-term care. Here, long-term care residents accounted for 81 per cent of all COVID-19 deaths; the average in other countries stood at 38 per cent. More than 9,650 staff members had become infected, representing 10 per cent of all virus cases in Canada. Nine of those workers had died.

The disaster rumbled under the radar until, that same month, the Canadian Armed Forces (CAF) released a report on five care homes in Ontario. The province had called on the military in April to help with the urgent staffing crisis—or, as the CAF put it, "to provide humanitarian relief and medical support." The resulting report, which matter-of-factly detailed the distressed state of five homes in the province, was both devastating and nauseating. At one home in Etobicoke, residents with COVID-19 were not isolated and staff were given inadequate PPE and the (false) impression that PPE didn't have to be changed between patients or rooms. New staff weren't trained. Many personal support workers (PSWs) at the home couldn't access supplies to properly care for the residents, and they feared for their jobs if they used too many. Expired medication stocked the shelves. Cockroaches and other insects, like flies and ants, infested at least two homes. At one, in North York, some residents hadn't been bathed for weeks. Military staff observed patients crying for help with no response from PSWs or nurses for anywhere between thirty minutes to over two hours. At the other, in Pickering, patients were left in bed wearing soiled diapers. Food and belongings were kept out of reach. Mattresses were placed on floors, and walkers were hidden to prevent residents with mobility issues from wandering.

Underfeeding, poor hygiene, and bed confinement were reported at several of the homes. At one, the smell of rotten food belched through the air. At others, evening shifts went completely unstaffed. Decontamination procedures often didn't exist or weren't followed. At a home in Brampton, PSWs didn't wash their hands between patients. Workers in many homes were under the same misconception as those in Etobicoke: PPE wasn't changed in between rooms, even when a resident was known to be COVID-positive; some wore scarves under their masks; equipment wasn't disinfected and neither were rooms. Across the board, staff burnout was rife. People were bone-tired. Some staff hadn't seen their families in months. In most cases, the lowered level of care wasn't intentionally cruel, or even wilfully subpar. The vast majority of PSWs were doing the best they could with little direction or training, even less protection, and severe shortages. A lot of them were being asked to perform nurses' duties beyond their skills or training. It was like trying to spread a tablespoon of jam over a dozen loaves of bread. As the CAF report noted, "The staffing is such that it is impossible to provide care at a pace that is appropriate to each resident or allow them any kind of independence."

The report was surprising, and it wasn't. Laura Bulmer is a PSW advocate, registered nurse, and a full-time professor at a community college in Ontario. At first, she didn't pay too much attention to the incoming pandemic—in fact, she "pooh-poohed" the virus at the beginning of 2020. She had, to put it lightly, other things to worry about. In July 2019, her younger sister died from ovarian cancer. Six months later, Bulmer herself was diagnosed with uterine cancer after contracting pneumonia. She had surgery to remove her tumours in January, then later left the city for her family lake house to recuperate. Once the WHO declared COVID-19 a pandemic,

Bulmer began to feel guilty for not being able to join the front line. She knew her health put her at sky-high risk levels, but she badly wanted to help. She wanted to be slogging it out with her fellow nurses. In April, she returned to work at her college—here she uses air quotes around "returned" because, really, she stayed at the lake house, working from her make-shift desk.

As she made her way from the summit of Email Mountain, she read note after note that made her "blood boil." More than most, Bulmer knew the challenges PSWs faced: endemic short-staffing and scant resources, depressingly low pay, suffocating pressure to perform care that wasn't in their job description and for which they hadn't trained. For her entire career, Bulmer had worked to give PSWs the recognition they deserved—she'd created dedicated career fairs at her college, lobbied governments, and become chair of the Canadian Association of Continuing Care Educators—all so they wouldn't be treated, as one former student put it during the pandemic, like "glo-rified shit cleaners." Bulmer knew it would be far, far too easy to scapegoat them for the burgeoning long-term care crisis. She decided she wouldn't let it happen. This was how she could help.

In May, she wrote an op-ed in *Maclean's* arguing that the national regulation of PSWs could have largely prevented the unfolding tragedy in long-term care facilities. The lack of stan-dardization puts workers, residents, and the general public at risk, she told me, starting with an inconsistency in training and education. Training can take place in a high school, a community college, or a private career college. If they wanted to, she added, anyone, with or without experience, could join the bogus ranks and start their own school for training PSWs, luring new Canadians with the promise of quick learning, and even quicker hiring—all for an exorbitant fee, of course. On top of this, there isn't a singular name to describe such care work. A person may be called a PSW or a care aide, or they may be called a clinical assistant, a certified health aide, a home attendant, an orderly, or, as Bulmer put it, "tens of other names." Attempting to standardize a profession that has no standard name can feel like a dog chasing its tail. Without such regulation, however, it isn't only training that can vary wildly, but also pay and contract terms. As a result, many PSWs work at several homes at once to make ends meet. A pandemic like COVID-19, or an epidemic like SARS, forces them to pick one job site, creating a domino effect of short staff. The result of all this is a workforce that is majority women, many of whom are racialized or new to Canada.

"We're talking about voiceless, vulnerable people looking after other voiceless, vulnerable people," said Bulmer. "And it's just a big shit show." Regulation would mean licensing, proper advocacy and ethics boards, and public registries. PSWs would commit to a professional code of ethics and standards of practice; so too would their employers. The public would be able to bring complaints and concerns forward to a professional college, which would, in turn, mete out discipline as necessary—a structure that exists for other professions that are responsible for the bulk of society's care, such as nurses, doctors, teachers, and so on. Bulmer believes standardization would also mitigate what she calls "scope creep," which can happen when overloaded facilities begin demanding PSWs do things for which they were never trained. Examples of this might be delegating a PSW to administer medication or change wound dressings, among other things, all of which require a level of medical assessment and are, incidentally, actions that the CAF reported being performed improperly. Bulmer and others have been advocating for regulation for at least fifteen years, stressing the benefits of all-around improved safety and care. If anything could nudge their dream closer to reality, it seemed—from the outside at least—like the pandemic might be it. As cases and deaths tallied higher and higher in care homes across the country, though, that isn't exactly what happened.

The same day Bulmer officially returned to work, she also saw an email from a company that wanted to create a six-to-eight-week online PSW course. She lost it. How could a truncated online course hope to safely and effectively teach students everything they needed? You can't change a person's sheets through a screen, learn how to feed them, lift an unwieldy body into a wheelchair. She also wondered how many companies would try to cash in on the shortage. Bulmer lost it again when Quebec announced its own in-person fast-track program to train an additional ten thousand PSWs for fall. She understood the need to replenish the workforce. Quebec had been slow to enforce a ban on working at multiple care homes, and as a result, the disease had spread fast. By May, around nine thousand PSWs in Quebec had either refused to work or had become sick with COVID-19. But Bulmer doubted the mass of new students could learn how to provide effective care in just a few months, no matter the urgent need. She, and others, also worried about the burden it would place on PSWs already in the field, who had to help train the thousands of new workers. None of this would have happened if PSWs were already regulated, she surmised. More than that, she didn't think a quick fix would *fix* anything. After all, the pandemic hadn't created the mess; it had only exacerbated it.

Fifty-one-year-old Arlene Reid died on April 27 while her daughter frantically performed CPR. Like many PSWs, Reid worked several jobs: one in home care, one in long-term care, and another in a retirement home. During the weeks before she caught COVID-19, none of them appeared to make her feel safe. Each had a shortage of PPE; her home care job provided two surgical masks every five days. It also took her to multiple locations, in and out of people's houses and apartments, and at least one of her patients, she'd been told, was tested for the virus. Reid lived with a daughter who was battling cancer. She didn't want to put her in danger, and besides, the government had told people to stay home, not zig-zag across the GTA. In March, she'd gone on a trip home to Jamaica and, after her mandated quarantine, was hesitant to return to work. She told her employers so. One pressured her to return anyway, or be labelled with job insubordination. Another considered her "resigned." So she went to the first and she worked, and on April 17 she felt unwell enough to get tested. On April 20, the results came back positive. Reid, who has five children and three grandchildren, moved out of the house with her ill daughter and into the house with the one who would watch her take her last breath.

Initially, Reid had a mild fever and a cough. As she became more sick, she developed a shortness of breath and a higher fever and began vomiting. She also experienced a loss of smell and taste. Through it all, she tried to stay positive, right to the end, telling that daughter, "I'm going to get better. Mommy is going to be okay. I'm going to walk away from this." And for a while, her daughters said, it did seem like she was getting better. After days of self-isolation in a bedroom inside the Brampton, Ontario, home, her cough had subsided. But the bad breathing stuck, until one night, feeling her condition rapidly decline, she asked her daughter to call 911. By the time the paramedics got there, it was too late. Officially, it's unknown where she contracted the virus, but her daughters believe it was through work. In addition to the home care, Reid worked at least one shift at one of the long-term care homes that required military support. Her employers, perhaps unsurprisingly, contend they are not to blame. Reid was the second PSW in Ontario to die from the virus, and the third healthcare worker. "My mom died at my house," her daughter told the *Globe and Mail*. "She just wanted to get better."

Gloria Turney woke up to a text about her friend's death at 5:30 a.m. the Monday morning Reid died. The two had grown up together in Jamaica, and Turney thought of her as more of a family member than a friend. Reid had immigrated to Canada before her, and they reconnected when Turney followed. Like Reid, Turney has been a PSW for twenty years, working in home and community care. Before the pandemic, her day started at 6 a.m. She'd take the bus to her clients' homes and help them get out of bed, get washed and dressed, make sure they took their medication, help them get their breakfast— whatever it was, Turney helped. On any given day, she might see up to eight people, travelling between homes or between rooms at a retirement building. A visit could take fifteen minutes, or it could take three hours. A work day could end in the afternoon or at 10 p.m. She liked travelling every day, the freedom it gave her, how easy it was to take a break and grab a coffee after a difficult client. As the virus spread through the province, though, Turney decided it was no longer safe to be a "busser." She requested to work at one location a twenty-minute ride away, a transitional bed facility, where people stay as they're awaiting a permanent long-term care spot. She was working there when the first PSW in Ontario died; Turney had reached out to their shared union and asked, "What's going on?" People were putting their lives on the line.

It was even worse when Reid died, fear and grief and shock folding together. Turney knew her; her family knew her. She hadn't heard about the death from the news, or from a co-worker, but from Reid's sister. It hit home harder. Now the cost of the disease had a face, shared laughter, a whole life of togetherness, love. She realized anybody could die from COVID-19. She realized she had to get up and go to work. Turney can't speak for what Reid's employers should have done. But she knows what she would have liked her company to do if the same awful, tragic, unthinkable thing had happened to her. *Say something.* Maybe the company doesn't want to admit fault. Fine. Turney just doesn't want to see them sweep a life, and a death, under the proverbial rug. The absolute bare minimum an employer can do is send condolence flowers, she added. And sure, she knows that some companies did, although mostly after Turney and her union "got loud" about the PSW deaths. What she'd have liked to see, though, is for any company that employs a worker who died to reach out to the family. To phone them. To get sincere about how truly, terribly sorry they are. To express care for the people they sent to the front line. "All these years of working with you," she said, "and a bouquet of flowers—is that it?"

Turney is, however, sadly used to the indifference, and even callousness, of companies toward workers. She's been part of her union's bargaining committee for years. For a decade, she's been lobbying for better pay and better treatment. In 2013, her union went on strike to protest the $14 hourly wage for PSWs. They walked away with less than a ten-cent increase. So, they pushed the government. As a result, the hourly wage was bumped to $19, where it was capped, and the increase was rolled out over a number of years. After five years at the $19 cap, Turney and her union went back to the government and the companies with a simple message: you need to do better. That time, they walked away with a thirty-two-cent wage increase, this time rolled out over three years. In 2020, Turney made $19.13 an hour. It will be 2022 before she sees $19.32. If she hadn't lived in the same place in Burlington for years, or if she ever lost it, she knows she wouldn't be able to afford rent in her city. She doesn't have a pension, and unless she works 1,352 hours in a year, she doesn't get benefits. This, she told me, is why PSWs work in so many different homes at once. It's why some of them quit when the pandemic hit; it's also why some of them couldn't afford to stop going to work. It's why patients' care and living conditions both suffer. The pandemic may have made the situation worse, Turney said, but it also made it unavoidable.

Suddenly, there was nowhere else to look, she told me. "This was the topic of the day—you had to look at it. Now your mothers, your fathers, your grandmothers are affected." People could no longer look away; they, too, now had a face to put to the problem, the grief, the fear. For Turney it could be frustrating to watch puppy-dog-eyed politicians act aghast, heartbroken. "We've been telling you for years that these are the conditions," she added. "We've been asking for years for you to help us to have a voice, and nobody chose to." Still, she does not regret working through the pandemic. For one, she loves her job. And second, she knows it helped her make it through the worst of the isolating time. She cannot imagine staying alone, inside her home, day after day. In March, she was supposed to go home to Jamaica. Her first vacation in six years would have been to see her sister, who had been diagnosed with Stage I breast cancer. In a normal year, she would have gone to visit her sick sister two or three times. Now, she had to settle for video calls. As much as she helped her clients through the pandemic, they helped her, too. They helped keep her mind off what should have been. Kept her from staying in her house alone. Gave her a purpose.

There is one client in particular who helped Turney make it through. A retired realtor, she, like Turney, was born in December. Turney describes her as witty, with a keen sense of humour. "Nothing you do bothers this woman," she said. If her body had been adjusted into an uncomfortable position by accident, she made a joke of it: "Okay, why don't you do that again?" If someone asked if she was good, she'd quip, "You know I'm always good." To Turney, she was the best. Sometimes they'd joke around so much that, through laughter, Turney would plead, "Behave yourself!" The woman's family would know when Turney was working because she would help her put on makeup before their FaceTime. Lipstick, blush, her brows—everything. She would go all out. They'd look inside the woman's jewellery box and find something to match her outfit. The funny thing is, added Turney, she herself hardly wears cosmetics at all, and certainly not every day. But she helped her client because that's what made her client feel whole, happy. Because that's what you do when you believe somebody, no matter their age, has the right to dignity, good care, and a fulfilling life.

In mid-March, a couple of days after the WHO declared a pandemic, the term "Boomer Remover" began trending on Twitter. It had, by then, appeared in more than sixty-five thousand tweets and references to the higher mortality rate among older people infected with COVID-19. The so-called joke riffed off the "OK Boomer" meme of earlier social media fame, and seemed to suggest that the deaths of those in one of the virus's more susceptible age ranges, fifty-six to seventy-four—a group whom younger generations often characterize as entitled, racist environment destroyers—maybe wasn't such a tragedy, after all. Around that same time, WHO director-general Tedros Adhanom Ghebreyesus slammed countries that were responding slowly, or poorly, to the virus because they believed it killed only senior or older people. To categorize, and then dismiss, the virus as merely a senior-killer, he added, represented "a moral decay of the society." In the *New York Times*, Dr. Louise Aronson questioned the constant use of the qualifier *only*—as if, she wrote, "COVID-19 didn't matter much if it was a scourge only among the old." Indeed, that seemed to be what hundreds, perhaps millions, of us thought.

For many politicians, media members, and, I'm embarrassed to say, those in my own social circles, the word *only* was breathed as a relief; it felt nearly as potent as a vaccine. It was a way to reassure, a way to say, barely between the lines, that *not everybody will survive this virus, but everybody who matters will.* Days into his country's lockdown, the lieutenant governor of Texas even suggested grandparents would be willing to sacrifice themselves for the country's economic future— a proposed solution that gained surprising ground in the U.S. Ultra-conservative talking head Ben Shapiro said, "If grandma dies in a nursing home at age 81, that's tragic and that's terrible, also the life expectancy in the United States is 80." (For the record, if somebody reaches eighty, they are expected to live at least another decade.) Ukraine's ex–health minister said those over aged sixty-five were already "corpses." All around the world, people acted as though, if the elderly died, well, too bad, but not really. All around the world, we called our grandmothers and our mothers and told them to stay inside.

Canada's own callous, ageist attitudes toward seniors didn't come with as much punditry as some countries', but that doesn't mean they didn't exist. We saw such attitudes in our early apathetic treatment of those who live in long-term care and in the mirrored treatment of those who cared for them. They materialized again when public discourse shifted around the virus after health officials and common sense each debunked the myths about who COVID-19 affected—yes, younger people can get sick; yes, they can die—often (but not always) making the threat "real" for many people. And we saw our attitudes exposed yet again when, despite the still-unique vulnerability of seniors—their mortality rate remains much higher, and more of them are hospitalized—health policy and collective grief both seemed to favour younger demographics. Take, for example, the observations of twenty researchers, many of them Canadian, who together asked difficult, uncomfortable questions about the ageism and discrimination exposed by our response to the pandemic. "It is revealing that the younger adults who have died from complications of COVID-19 throughout the world have often generated long and in-depth media reports," wrote the authors, "while the deaths of thousands of older adults have been simply counted and summarized, if they were documented at all."

As a result, thousands of women's deaths were reduced to a statistic. What's more, unlike in other countries, where men account for a greater portion of COVID-19 deaths, the sheer number of long-term care deaths here has tipped the gender balance during the first wave—largely because women comprise a larger share of residents in such facilities across Canada. We've been asked to care about their deaths because they could have been our mothers or grandmothers, sweet ladies with cotton-candy hair, flower-scented skin, and kind words. Follow that same logic, and you're asking someone to care about sexual violence because it could happen to your sisters, daughters, mothers. In both cases, we should care about these women not because of who they were to *us*, or what gender role they can be neatly categorized into, but because of who *they* are: extraordinary humans. Ageism would have us believe that most of these women were doddering around in their homes, knitting doilies, drooling, and waiting for death. It would have us believe that their value to society had passed. Beyond being morally reprehensible, those perceptions simply aren't true. Many senior women volunteer in the communities and in their care centres. They teach younger generations and pass down wisdom. They're caretakers and creators. And, in many cases, they were trailblazers.

Thelma Coward-Ince was one such woman. In April, she contracted COVID-19 inside her Halifax long-term care home, Northwood. At the time, the facility accounted for most of the province's virus-related deaths. By the next month, long-term care deaths would encompass 97 per cent of all deaths in Nova Scotia. And by June, fifty-three residents at Northwood had died from the virus. Each of them had life stories. Coward-Ince herself graduated from Mount Saint Vincent University with a bachelor of arts. At sixteen, she began working and, shortly after, joined the Royal Canadian Navy, where she knocked down a domino of firsts. She was the first Black naval reservist and the first Black senior secretary as chief of staff to the admiral. At the National Defence, she was the first Black manager and the only female manager in her unit for more than a decade—there were also fewer than one hundred women working out of a total two thousand members in the division. She served on multiple boards, too, including the Black United Front, the Health Association of African Canadians, the Canadian Ethnocultural Council, and the Nova Scotia Advisory Commission on AIDS. And for twenty years, until she was diagnosed with dementia, she sang with the Nova Scotia Mass Choir.

Northwood's first outbreak was considered resolved as of July 2020, around the same time the rest of the country's COVID-19 case counts plummeted. Mere months later, however, the country's second wave began to crest—and it looked like Canada might fail its elderly again. By fall, cases began to reappear in long-term care centres, including in some that had previously quelled their outbreaks. The facility where Roisin O'Brien worked was one of them. By October, resident cases in Ontario long-term care homes were approaching April numbers at 159 virus-positive patients; at 199, staff cases had already surpassed their April tallies. The province asked the Red Cross to help in several homes, just as the disaster relief organization had done over the summer in Quebec. It was as if the July and August heat had evaporated caution, community regard, and maybe also a little bit of the fear. It also seemed to erase much of the mass outpouring of support for frontline and essential workers, and with it the pressure to better protect them. As the quarantine ended, PSWs were largely forgotten. "Two months ago, we were heroes," Turney told me toward the end of August. "When have you last heard that?"

———

On O'Brien's sixth or seventh day of working on the COVID-19 floor, infections specialists from Vancouver Coastal Health visited the centre where she worked. On the day they arrived, the facility was, as had become the new normal, short-staffed. As O'Brien listened to a lecture on proper PPE use, she became more and more upset. Then, she exploded. "We need people," she told them. "We need bodies." She peppered them with questions: Are you a nurse? Are you a care aid? Can you work? People were dying, and she knew there were not enough people at the facility anymore to properly take care of them. What did it matter if staff knew the proper precautions if there was nobody there to follow them? "I lost it," O'Brien said. "I burst out into tears." She had to leave the room. She came back, of course; there were only two other care aides working the shift with her. She wasn't about to leave them alone. She wasn't about to leave anybody alone. Especially the people who were dying. "There was not one person who died alone," she added. "I made sure of that."

When she knew somebody wasn't doing well, she'd make sure to monitor them. Every half hour, she'd stop her work, go in and check on them, hold their hand, satisfy herself that they were okay. Then she'd run back to whatever she was doing. Then, thirty minutes and back again. She'd do this for everybody whose health had stuttered, looping from person to person, never leaving anybody alone for too long. If her check-in revealed they were getting worse, she'd stay and wait. If it was the end—thirteen people died during the first outbreak and eighty-nine became sick—she'd make sure they didn't face it alone. It was better, she said, when a person had family in the city, or nearby. O'Brien could call them and they could come in, dressed in full PPE. They were better good-byes, and she could feel the weight lift off her when a person's son or daughter sat at their bedside, whispering love and reassurance. Not everybody had family left, though, and for those times, O'Brien was there. It wasn't always peaceful, like in the movies. People call out, they get restless, they do not want to go. O'Brien, who had already seen so much death in her job, felt the sharp difference of dying in a pandemic. "It was so many people in such a short amount of time," she said. "It was just continual, continual, continual—I didn't have time to process it."

She wasn't on the COVID-19 floor for too long before she, too, got sick. Her swab test for the virus came back negative, but O'Brien knew there was no way she should keep work-ing. She felt like she had a terrible cold; she felt like she had the virus. By that time, she said, some of the care aides who'd originally tested positive were finishing their quarantines and able to come back to work—"It was almost like we were swap-ping places." O'Brien eventually took a total of four COVID-19 tests, with each coming back negative. However, she also knew that sometimes the tests give a false negative, meaning they indicate you don't have the virus when you do. The reported rate of false negatives ranges between 2 and 37 per cent. A later antibody test, which uses a person's blood and can show whether they had the virus in the past, came back positive. O'Brien returned to work after about ten days of self-isolation. By that time, she was able to go back to her regular floor, a piece of good news mitigated by the fact that the virus was now on every floor. At least it was now easier to sequester virus-positive patients in their rooms. Easier to stop the spread.

O'Brien doesn't see herself changing her job any time soon. Yes, it's hard. Yes, it's scary. Yes, it isn't for everybody. But she knows that, at the end of the day, she can go home. Her clients *are* home. And, as the daughter of two nurses, she sees it as her duty to help people. To make connections with them. To make their lives better. She wants people to know that a lot of PSWs feel that way—even the ones who got sick, even the ones who, for many reasons, could not work during the pandemic. At her facility, and many others, the staff who were left did the best that they could. It wasn't that they were all incompetent, or that they didn't care. They just didn't have the magical power to manifest being in a dozen places at once. They couldn't raise the funding for better staffing, supplies, or conditions. It would have been infinitely, unimaginably worse if even a fraction fewer of the PSWs who staffed facilities, homes, and community care across the country weren't there. Think about that for a second. We know it was bad, and it could have been *worse*. When I spoke to O'Brien before the second wave in the fall and the re-emergence of the virus in her facility, she worried about what would happen if companies and government didn't use the infection lull to shore up resources at care homes. "If something like this happens again," she warned, "the whole system is going to fall apart." Along with everyone inside it.

"WHEN WE DECIDE THAT WE, AS HUMAN BEINGS, ARE THE PRIORITY, EVERYTHING ELSE WILL FOLLOW FROM THAT DECISION."

Paulette Senior,
President and CEO of the
Canadian Women's Foundation

Nine

RECOVERY

Alyson Kelvin cannot simply walk into her Containment Level 3 lab at VIDO-InterVac. First, she enters a locker room, where she changes from her regular street clothes into her scrubs. Then, she enters a secure hallway and a room nicknamed the "clean" change room. There, she preps everything she'll need to work with that day and changes again into a new pair of scrubs—these ones only go into the lab. Afterward, she enters the "dirty" change room. That's where she'll put on all her equipment: special socks, double gloves, and her Tyvek coverall suit. The effect is half marshmallow, half spacesuit. She'll also put on a hood and helmet that are equipped for filtered air circulation via a hose that hangs from the back of her head like a ponytail and clips into a power pack. The pack feeds the clean, virus-free air and sits around her waist. To Kelvin, the air that flows through the suit is icy, and she usually layers two long-sleeved shirts under her scrubs. Once inside her lab, which, incidentally, she can see into from a square window in her office, the real work begins—that is, helping to build a vaccine that millions see as their road back to normalcy, their quick salvation, and the end point of the global pandemic that drastically, almost incomprehensibly, changed the world.

Every vaccine has the same starting point, said Kelvin. First, you have to know what the pathogen is—not such an easy task with an emerging virus, or a mutating one. After the virus is sequenced, however, the question of how to develop a vaccine, and which type is the best, can have multiple answers. As Kelvin put it, "Vaccines teach your immune system what to be ready for." And the lesson can change depending on the virus or bacteria. While every vaccine itself is pathogen-specific, there are several different approaches to getting there, each known as a vaccine platform. The most common and historically used ones are called classic platforms.

One such immune system prepper is called a live attenuated vaccine—when the virus itself can be weakened and used. Live attenuated vaccines have been employed to fend off everything from the rotavirus to measles, mumps, and rubella. Another long-chosen germ-fighting method, the inactivated vaccine, starts with a killed version of the virus or bacteria. The polio shot, flu shot, and hepatitis A vaccine all fall under this classic platform. If a weakened or deactivated version of the pathogen cannot be used, a virologist might instead break apart the virus or bacteria to use different pieces of it, including its protein, sugar, or capsid. Subunit vaccines, for example, contain only the antigenic parts of a pathogen—their unique protein or glycol-protein markers. Sometimes, these antigens stay the same, and sometimes, like with the flu virus, they mutate (which is why a new flu vaccine must be developed and disseminated every year). Then there are toxoid vaccines, like the tetanus shot, which, as the name suggests, use the toxins produced by certain bacteria to elicit immunity in a person's body.

Health Canada approved its first COVID-19 vaccine, developed by Pfizer-BioNTech, on December 9, 2020. A few weeks later, on December 23, it approved its second, this one developed by Moderna. By January 2021, the federal government secured access to 80 million doses, with the opportunity to buy more of both, if needed. The first shipments of each began arriving that same month. Both vaccines need two doses to be effective, and while both also require cold storage, Pfizer's only remains stable at a bone-chilling -70 degrees Celsius—preventing it from being shipped to certain remote Canadian communities that lacked capacity to store it. Such limitations are some of the reasons why researchers don't stop developing vaccines after the first one works. Plus, we have an entire planet to vaccinate, and need a whole lot of shots to do it. Unique restrictions exist the world over.

As of mid-October 2020, the WHO estimated there were 198 SARS-CoV-2 vaccines in development worldwide, with 44 of them already in clinical evaluation. Many of them, like most of the vaccines currently in use worldwide, are using classic platforms. "However," as a July 2020 article in *Nature Materials* noted, "certain limitations are associated with several of these platforms that make them less amenable to fast vaccine production in a pandemic." Some would require growing massive quantities of SARS-CoV-2; others, extensive testing for safe use. Neither option is especially attractive when thousands of people are dying and an entire planet has been put on pause. That's why, when it comes to SARS-CoV-2, many researchers quickly began developing solutions under next-generation platforms that have, to date, not been widely used on humans. While they come with their own potential pitfalls—namely, that they haven't been around long enough to be tested for long-term safe and effective use—they can be developed on a significantly truncated timeline and are generally easier to manufacture on the necessary millions-plus scale. These competing risks and benefits are another reason why scientists are tackling the vaccine solution from numerous angles and not putting all their needles in one biohazardous bucket. In her first year at VIDO-Intervac, Kelvin worked on three different platforms at once, two of which point to the possible future of vaccines—that is, if the world keeps producing possible global pandemics, which it sadly seems likely to.

One such next-gen platform is called a viral vector-based vaccine, which is based off the same platform as the Canadian-made Ebola vaccine. They work by inserting an incomplete segment of genetic material from the pathogen in question into a harmless virus that doesn't cause disease. Inside the body, this Frankensteined genetic material is then translated into proteins that activate the immune system response. This type of vaccine is also highly immunogenic, meaning one dose is often enough to do the trick. The other newer models that have risen to prominence in the fight against COVID-19 are called genetic platforms, which, as the name suggests, use a virus's own DNA or RNA to deliver the genetic template for a pathogen's antigens into the body. Both the Pfizer and Moderna shots are messenger RNA (mRNA) vaccines, which essentially send a harmless "recipe" for making coronavirus spike into our bodies, prepping our immune system response. Similarly, the vaccine Kelvin is working on uses the DNA for the coronavirus spike. Once inside the human body, it travels into a person's cells, which in turn start making spike, allowing immune cells to learn what it looks like and to elicit antibodies. Those prepared antibodies are then ready to encapsulate and bind around SARS-CoV-2 when it enters the body, blocking it from infection and effectively neutralizing the virus. Think of it as a microscopic game of "Say Uncle."

Genetic vaccines offer one big advantage: once the solution is cracked, they can be produced very quickly and at high, consistent quality. That's because the genetic strands used in the vaccine can be made synthetically, based on viral sequence information alone. In other words, manufacturers don't have to worry about their ability to culture the virus. That isn't the case for the third vaccine Kelvin is working on, which is a protein-based vaccine. With it, researchers are again using a spike-targeted approach. The spikes they've created are noninfectious; the rest of the disease isn't there—think, a toothless vampire. Again, once the isolated spike is inside the body, it will learn what the protein looks like and have a jump-start on its defence. These types of vaccines carry their own unique risk, as there is no guarantee that immunological memory will be formed for future response. They take longer to produce. That's because virologists actually need to make the protein themselves, taking the time to culture cells in a lab. They then have to purify it and run quality control to make sure it can be injected into somebody and do what it's meant to. In each case, Kelvin uses an animal susceptible to SARS-CoV-2—this time, ferrets—to evaluate the vaccine candidates and conduct a battery of tests. She knows a vaccine is on the right track once the ferret is completely protected and can no longer be infected with the virus.

A lot of people have asked Kelvin if she does feel pressured to, well, save the world. It isn't that she feels no pressure at all, she told me, but mostly she just feels like she has to do her job. "It's what I do," she added. "I was trained to do this. It's almost automatic." She knows that there are many vaccine researchers out there, and if her vaccines aren't the ones that ultimately make it into production, one or many of theirs will. Those researchers are learning from her, and she is also learning from them. All around the globe, women are showing up and doing their jobs, putting their brilliance and their collective brain power toward ending the pandemic. So, Kelvin will keep showing up to work, too. She'll put on all her protective gear every morning, and at the end of the day, she'll take it all off again. Afterward, from the "dirty" side, she'll place her scrubs in an autoclave—which she described as a "big sanitation oven"—and take them out from the "clean" side, where they're then washed and put back into circulation. She'll go to her hotel room and eat and read medical research and call her family. Eventually, in August, they will join her in Saskatoon, where they'll live for a year. And every day, she'll keep doing her part to return the world to normal.

In April, Cecie Elnicki agreed to participate in two possible upcoming COVID-19 vaccine trials. She'd previously volun- teered with the same company conducting the trials, Manna Research, for a potential vaccine against the dangerous, hospital-acquired Clostridioides difficile, or C. difficile, bac- teria, and also, a few years before that, for both a shingle vaccine and a flu vaccine. The media attention that followed her decision seemed to surprise her. One of her daughters was a frontline health worker during SARS, and the same daugh- ter's husband was now working in a critical care unit. They were doing their bit during the pandemic. This was her way of doing hers. She didn't see herself as a hero, and despite some interviewers' attempts to push her to say otherwise, she didn't see her decision as dangerous, either. She saw it as a sign of hope—and as a way to further medical progress. She thought back to her C. difficile trial and how it could save lives. She was only too glad to say yes again, but also, she stressed, it wasn't that big of a deal. Elnicki joked that she only shared a single concern when contacted: after hearing that one of the candidates came from the U.S., she quipped, "It doesn't have any disinfectant in it, does it?"

For all her modesty, people like Elnicki are a vital part of vaccine development, and especially so when that development is unlike anything previously attempted. Public health experts and virologists both widely agree the pandemic won't end until we have a vaccine. But what that means is more complex than many might realize. Under non-pandemic circumstances, vaccine development takes years, or even decades, making it an expensive, painstaking process. Attrition is high, and multiple candidates are often discarded before a vaccine is licensed for use in humans. Because of this, developers usually obey a set of established steps, checks, and balances, all in the same precise order. After animal trials are complete, human ones begin, following three distinct phases. The first vaccinates a small group of healthy people, who are monitored for adverse reactions. If the vaccine passes the first phase, it will next be administered to hundreds of subjects, where it will be evaluated for efficacy. The final phase stretches the net out to thousands, tracking participants to find out what happens when they naturally come into contact with the pathogen and determining whether it works at a group level. And not only does the vaccine have to work, it has to have the ability to be mass manufactured, all without losing quality or pushing the price point too high.

The slow and patient progress of these tried-and-tested steps, however, makes little sense in a pandemic. That's why researchers worldwide developed a new paradigm under SARS-CoV-2. They wouldn't dare skip steps—a certain disaster—but they decided they could do them all at once, without waiting to see if the traditional first step was successful. For example, in some cases, animal trials and phase 1 clinical trials have been happening in parallel. Kelvin, for instance, has continued her animal testing to determine the various candidates' safety and efficacy, even as her colleagues have sought government approval to begin human trials on some of those platforms, or have already started on others. In certain instances, developers also began early manufacturing scale-up and commercial scale processes before ascertaining whether the vaccine had concrete clinical proof of concept. Such concurrent work is undertaken at considerable financial risk; if a vaccine fails a step, the sunk cost may be much, much higher than usual. Complicating it all further, most of the next-generation platforms have never been licensed for use against any pathogen and, therefore, have never been manufactured at a large scale. Meaning, not only are vaccine developers taking a chance on whether the platform is viable, they're also taking a chance on whether it can be made on a significant scale. And even after all these problems are solved, countries still have to convince enough people to get the vaccine.

Though they've saved lives and helped control, and even eradicate, disease for centuries, vaccines have never had an easy or straight narrative. In 1717, Lady Mary Wortley Montagu, the wife of the British ambassador to Turkey, witnessed her first variolation in Constantinople. A precursor to vaccination, the process involved inserting a thread into the pustule of a person infected with a mild case of smallpox, and then inserting that saturated thread into a small cut in the arm of a healthy person, where it was left to soak for twenty-four hours. The motivation behind the experimental procedure was simple: everyone seemed to know that if a person survived smallpox, they never became infected with it again. So why not try to induce a mild, survivable case to ward off a more serious one? At the time, this method of protecting against smallpox—a disease that could both kill and permanently disfigure—was common in the Middle East and Asia, but not in Lady Montagu's home continent of Europe. As someone who'd survived but been gravely scarred by the disease, she vowed to have her children undergo variolation. When it worked, she spread the gospel upon her return to England. The apparently miraculous procedure was, however, met with plenty of skepticism, and it was initially carried out only on prisoners, who were offered freedom if they survived. Eventually, the method gained advocates across the Western world. George Washington used it to inoculate his entire army. Catherine the Great tried it, and the Princess of Wales inoculated her daughters. The controversy stuck, though: variolation was expensive, and it risked both killing its recipients and further spreading the disease.

Still, the process undoubtedly inspired Edward Jenner, who is frequently dubbed the "father of vaccination." Working as a rural doctor in England, Jenner noticed that milkmaids infected with cowpox, a mild illness, also seemed to gain immunity to smallpox. Though he wasn't the first to notice the seeming coincidence, he was the first to document it and to gather data to confirm it. And, in 1796 he convinced his gardener to let him experiment on the man's eight-year-old son. (Eighteenth-century England may have been the peak of new science, but it was evidently not so great on the ethics front.) Jenner first gave the boy the cowpox virus, and then smallpox. He called his new process a "vaccination," drawing from the Latin word *vaccinus*, meaning "from cows," and thus naming the method after the black-and-white spotted animals that had made it possible. The smallpox vaccine came with less risk than variolation, and Jenner quickly gained high-profile converts, including Pope Pius VII and Napoleon, as well as high-profile controversy.

Indeed, the birth of vaccines arrived with a twin: the birth of the anti-vaccination movement. In part, Jenner did some of the damage himself. He refused, even in the face of good evidence, to admit his vaccine did not offer lifelong immunity. (Today, it's believed the smallpox vaccine lasts up to twenty years before a person has to be revaccinated.) But opposition also came in the form of libertarianism: people resented the apparent intruding powers of the state, under what they saw as the guise of public health measures—call it, perhaps, the great, great, great, great grandparent to the current anti-mask movement. Others feared it violated God and nature to put something from a cow inside a human. As Frank M. Snowden wrote in *Epidemics and Society*, cartoons depicting vaccine recipients as hapless horn-sprouting monsters began to rise in popularity. One doctor stoked the hysteria, added Snowden, by saying women who took the vaccine would wander into fields and embark on sexual relations with bulls. Nonetheless, Jenner's smallpox vaccine marched on over the next two centuries and, in 1980, the WHO declared victory over the virus. Thanks to a concerted public health effort and vaccines themselves, naturally occurring smallpox was wiped from the earth.

But the anti-vaccination movement persisted. Less than two decades after smallpox was eliminated, British surgeon Andrew Wakefield published a since-debunked article in the *Lancet* that linked the measles, mumps, and rubella vaccine to autism-spectrum disorders. It didn't seem to matter that biological signs of autism are readily visible in utero, or that it was later discovered that he'd knowingly fabricated the medical histories of his subjects, or even that he accepted six hundred thousand dollars from a law firm planning to sue vaccine manufacturers. As Joshua S. Loomis sharply noted in *Epidemics*, "Suddenly, everyone was an infectious disease expert because they had read a secondhand account of a study on a blog or website." It was, as Loomis put it, "an explosion of ignorance." Once rare, measle outbreaks began reoccurring, and have continued to do so. Whooping cough was under control for decades, something that is no longer true. The scrutiny and misinformation campaign surrounding the human papillo-mavirus (HPV) vaccine has allowed the virus to stick around. The more resistance there is to the idea of preventable disease, the more opportunity said diseases have to evolve. The anti-vaccine movement has the same potential to damage efforts against COVID-19. In October 2020, for example, *Nature Medicine* released a survey of people in nineteen countries that showed only 71.5 per cent said they would be very or somewhat likely to take a COVID-19 vaccine. The rest said they would hesitate or outright refuse. It's just enough for herd immunity in Canada, but it's still distressing—especially since a December 2020 survey of Canadians showed only 48 per cent would immediately roll up their sleeves for a shot. (It was, at least, a welcome 8 per cent rise from the month before.) As those such as Kelvin and Elnicki do their parts, it will still be up to the rest of us to do ours.

If vaccines are the nuclear bomb in the fight against COVID-19, antivirals are the infantry. Unfortunately, though, viral illnesses are notoriously harder to treat than bacterial infections. In fact, after the discovery of penicillin in 1945, it took nearly another forty years for the first antiviral drug to be licensed. As noted earlier, pathogenic bacteria are largely free-living, single-celled organisms. That means antibiotics can target bacteria cells within the body while leaving our own cells unharmed. Viruses, on the other hand, are gifted hijackers that use our own cells to replicate themselves. Because of this, it's difficult to stop their reproduction without harming the host. While certain antibiotics can treat a wide variety of bacterial infections, antivirals are usually limited to a single virus, or a virus group. The first licensed antiviral, aciclovir, was introduced in the 1970s and treated herpesvirus infections, including cold sores and chickenpox. Like a virus, aciclovir is tricky, camouflaging itself as a nucleoside, the building block of DNA. Essentially, it terminates viral DNA replication and spares uninfected host cells. The crew of HIV antiviral drugs, taken together, is another example of a working, established drug therapy. The flu can also be treated with antivirals that inhibit the virus and block its entry into host cells. And, as Canada registered record-breaking case counts and the U.S. watched its own case count climb unabated in October, the latter country approved the first COVID-19 drug. Remdesivir is an antiviral that can cut recovery times by five days. It was a big breakthrough, but it wasn't the only one.

Throughout the end of 2019 and early 2020, immunologist Eleanor Fish was, as usual, travelling abroad. At each conference or academic institution, she shared the same message. "The twentieth century was the century of bacteria, and then along came antibiotics," she told me. "The twenty-first century is going to be one of viral infections." So, she'd asked the gathered experts, how are we going to handle this? How are we going to prepare ourselves? Closer to home, the U of T professor and scientist at the Toronto General Hospital Research Institute would share another, additional warning: Canada is a lightning rod for viral outbreaks. Our wonderfully diverse population means that people will arrive at our border from all around the world. They will cross it, in both directions, by plane, boat, train, car, and some of them, sometimes, will bring a virus with them. It doesn't matter where the outbreak originates, added Fish. When it stops moving, the chances are it will end up here, where it will spread. Because of all this, she thinks it is a lost cause to keep developing pathogen-specific antivirals. "You're always playing catch-up," she explained. A virus will travel, mutate, adapt, develop resistant strains—all of it often outpacing human speed. As an example, she pointed to Tamiflu, or oseltamivir, which many countries, including Canada, stockpiled in 2009 to fight the H1N1 swine flu pandemic. Canada recorded its first case on April 26, 2009, and its first aseltamivir-resistant case scant weeks later on July 21, 2009. It is not inconceivable that remdesivir could meet a similar fate. Which is why Fish argues it's time to stop making pathogen-specific drugs and try something else: interferons.

Interferons are a set of proteins that already occur naturally within our bodies. Our immune system cells secrete them in response to viruses and other threats. Discovered in 1957, interferons can be grouped into several classes that, together, help regulate the body's immune system response. They can, as the name suggests, interfere with viral proliferation, enhance innate or acquired immune system responses, and also respond to cancerous growth. When it comes to viruses like SARS-CoV-2, an infected cell may release interferons, stimulating nearby cells into entering an antiviral state. In other words, interferons won't kill a virus directly, but they will trigger a defence response in other cells, preventing the virus from replicating within them. This will, in turn, stem infection—sort of like turning each healthy cell into a battle fortress. Their use as a pharmaceutical product is not new. Since the 1980s, they've already been used to treat everything from Ebola to multiple sclerosis, to varying, and not always remarkable, effect. Fish herself has been studying their applications for decades. She has long believed that they do have a "wow factor" but that scientists have also missed interferons' true calling: as the perfect first responders in a global pandemic.

In December 2019, as news of the emerging novel coronavirus trickled out of Wuhan, Fish contacted colleagues in China who immediately set up an exploratory study using interferons to treat virus patients at a hospital in Wuhan. She was glad, but not exactly surprised, to discover the interferon treatment worked. Between January 16 and February 20, doctors administered interferon treatment to a total of seventy-seven people at the Union Hospital, Tongji Medical College at the Huazhong University of Science and Technology. The patients presented with a moderate case of COVID-19, and although they had been admitted into the intensive care unit, they did not require supplemental oxygen; it was early on into their possible disease progression. Researchers defined viral clearance as two consecutive negative tests at least twenty-four hours apart. Results were significant. Interferon treatment had accelerated viral clearance by approximately seven days. That's even faster than remdesivir, noted Fish. The treatment also reduced inflammatory markers of the disease. "Interferons are a no-brainer," she added.

Fish and her colleagues' study was published in May 2020 in *Frontiers in Immunology*. The publication had an oddly dual outcome: she became incredibly busy and optimistic, and also incredibly frustrated. When we spoke months later in early August, she joked that when she "allows" her iPhone to give her notifications, she will receive constant emails and calls from around the globe, from 7:30 a.m. until 11 p.m. She has helped researchers worldwide map out clinical trials, craft journal publications, edit research papers, and learn about interferon treatment. She has been asked, and has sometimes agreed, to join the scientific advisory boards of several pharmaceutical companies. She's given dozens of media interviews, everywhere. In short, she's made herself available around the clock. But even as she's seen interest in interferons explode, she's also seen a blanket of apathy.

If interferons were on, say, a dating app for antivirals, they'd have a lot going for them to make a person swipe right: they're already FDA approved, they have three decades of clinical experience, and they can work on a wide number of viruses—all of which also makes them an economically sound choice. Unfortunately, they have also not been very effective in their main use to date, which is against chronic virus infections. In that context, they work just "okay" and can have side effects that are "really quite unpleasant," said Fish. (It may be worth noting here that Fish is British by birth, and has the exact dry humour you might expect from a British scientist.) She knows that's why, even in the face of increasingly positive evidence, some scientists have been hesitant to throw them at another challenge. Luckily, that reticence had already started to shift when we spoke, thanks in large part to her persistence. Early on in the pandemic, she had, for example, shared her findings with the United States' Dr. Anthony Fauci, who, as Fish put it, "passed it on to his team, where it died a nice death." She noted, though, that it had since been resurrected, and that a randomized control trial was finally underway, too, which would only add to the growing body of evidence. And Fish thought fondly of her colleagues around the world who emailed her with their own disbelief as researchers scrambled to develop an antiviral, overlooking the one that already existed, and worked.

"Until there are organizations independent of Eleanor Fish who say, 'Yes, this looks promising,'" she noted, "This is going to be an uphill battle that continues." Still, Fish is used to proving people wrong. In 2014, she ran an interferon trial in Guinea to treat Ebola; the virus has more than a 60 per cent fatality rate in the country. Despite established protocol and recommendations, she refused to make it a randomized control trial; she believed the interferons would work and did not want to "randomize people to death." In the end, she convinced everybody there was enough historical data to provide an accurate contrast between those who received the treatment and those who didn't. And that contrast was stark: 67 per cent of the interferon-treated patients were still alive three weeks after infection, while only 19 per cent of those who received the standard care survived at day twenty-one. The study was so successful, she's now helping local health authorities develop an interferon clinic. Beneath all the frustration, COVID-19 offers a chance to prove naysayers wrong again. In the process, Fish won't only be helping us make it more safely through this pandemic—she'll be showing us how to better survive the next one.

Recovery is a complex thing. It goes deeper than vaccines and antivirals, further than containing SARS-CoV-2. It encapsulates the economy, human rights, housing, social resources, health care, what we demand from our governments, and what we'll no longer tolerate. Past pandemics spurred revolution and religion, squashed civilizations, and forked the course of history again and again and again. This pandemic is equally unlikely to fade quietly, returning the planet to 2019 in a great time-travel machine. Certainly, many people hope that it doesn't. Paulette Senior, the president and CEO of the Canadian Women's Foundation, is one of them. Of course, like all of us, she wants COVID-19 to stop. But as 2020 raged on, she also began to see the pandemic's possibility as a Great Reset. Watching how quickly society pivoted, all over the world, gave her hope. What she saw is that when all of our lives are at risk, humanity is capable of doing better. When it matters—and so many things still matter, from stopping domestic violence to fighting anti-Black racism to creating income equality—we can change. "All the old excuses of how difficult it would be to do this and that went out the window," said Senior. "And instead we could let in some fresh air."

Senior has spent much of her life tackling systemic barriers, particularly for women and girls. She's worked in social services, focusing on Toronto's most underserved neighbourhoods. She's managed shelters and employment programs and was the CEO of YWCA Canada for more than a decade. Her experiences when she was a young child as a newcomer from Jamaica to Canada also exposed her to her own set of systemic barriers. Which is to say, she has spent more than thirty years pushing for change and then the pandemic reaffirmed to her that such change can happen. We can transform in a heartbeat. It isn't about what's possible or impossible any longer, she told me. It's about: What kind of world are we committed to building? And, what kind of choices are we making when it comes to those whom the pandemic has most disastrously affected? If the pandemic has shown us that everything can come undone in an instant, it's also shown us that everything can be remade. We've seen unprecedented death and struggle, but we've also seen unprecedented kindness, leadership, support, and breathtaking innovation. We've seen that we're not stuck with what we have. So when we rebuild, argued Senior, why not rebuild something better—something that is in the best interest of all of us, and not just some? She has many ideas about what that could include: universal child care; inclusive, robust education that tells history from a more truthful perspective; a policing system that protects everybody and doesn't cost billions; committed, non-divisive politicians; "When we decide that we, as human beings, are the priority," she added, "everything else will follow from that decision."

Under that hopeful, adamant perspective—that we can build better—the Canadian Women's Foundation has released a series of research papers on building a better normal. Other women's organizations have joined them in their vision for a new Canada. For example, Senior's former organization, YWCA Canada, and the Institute for Gender and the Economy at the University of Toronto's Rotman School of Management jointly released a feminist economic recovery plan in July 2020. In it, they outlined eight "non-negotiable" steps the country should take to generate future prosperity, for everybody. Like Senior, the report's authors also saw hope in the broad range of people across Canada who, perhaps for the first time ever, realized things needed to change. To them, it looked like a necessary, and also encouraging, paradigm shift. They also recognized what many others, from PSWs to community leaders, had already stressed: COVID-19 alone isn't what broke us. "It took a pandemic for the country to see what was already broken," wrote the authors. "We cannot ignore the historical context that has created the unstable foundation for the harms we are seeing play out in this current crisis."

If Canada wanted not simply to recover what's been lost but to ensure well-being for decades to come, argued the report's authors, it needed to learn from the pandemic. After all, the recession itself was unlike anything the country had ever seen before; the solution needed to be equally ground-shaking. First, the joint plan outlined, the government would need to adopt an intersectional framework. To do so, it needed an unflinching account of the pandemic's consequences across race, age, gender identity, gender expression, disability, socio-economic status, sexual orientation, and immigration status—something that, nearly a year into the pandemic, it had not yet done. Second, after it had gathered better, more equitable data, it needed to follow that data and address the root cause of systemic racism. For instance, only $305 million, or less than 1 per cent of the federal government's COVID-19 funding, went to Indigenous communities; new economic stimulus couldn't follow the same flawed path. Jointly, it needed to address things like paid sick leave, safe housing, and other social determinants of health—and it would have to listen to the affected communities to figure out how to fix them. Third, the federal government needed to recognize that care work—both paid and unpaid—is essential, and then begin treating it as such. Meaning, better pay, more support, benefits, and better conditions. Meaning, universal child care.

Next up is investing in "good jobs" for people who don't traditionally have them: people of colour, trans people, the disabled. A "good job," added the authors, doesn't mean whatever stereotypical, classist thing you think it does; it means anything that is stable and provides a livable income. Fifth, the government would need to fight what's been dubbed the "shadow pandemic"—that is, the enormous rise in hate and violence, including, but definitely not limited to, domestic violence. As the recovery report noted, one in five Indigenous women told the Native Women's Association of Canada that they have experienced physical or psychological violence since the start of the pandemic. Chantel Moore, an Indigenous woman living in New Brunswick, and Regis Korchinski-Paquet, a Black-Indigenous woman living in Toronto, were killed during police wellness checks that took place during the first wave. And in June, the Vancouver Police Department said there had been a 600 per cent increase in reports of hate crimes against Asian communities. Prosperity shouldn't thrive in hate and violence, stressed the authors. Sixth, any recovery plan must also centre small businesses as well as business owners in underrepresented groups—like Alèthe Kaboré and Sarah Taher. Both of these categories represent significantly untapped economic potential. Seventh, the government must provide the infrastructure to make it all happen: housing, clean water, broadband access. The new economy won't succeed if people can't access the foundations. Lastly, wrote the authors, any decision-making must include diverse voices. "To ensure an equitable recovery," stressed the report, "we need to shift whose knowledge is valued in the conversation."

It's an ambitious plan, but the women of the pandemic have already provided the blueprint. Their work has shown us the way forward—and it's exposed the unconscionable pitfalls we must avoid as we move past COVID-19. This book has never been about perfection. The women you've met have revealed astonishing strength, and they've suffered immeasurable loss. They've made their own mistakes, and they've borne the brunt of others'. But what they all have in common is that, during the worst time in contemporary society, they tried. They tried to connect us. They tried to keep us safe. They tried to look out for each other. They tried to keep us healthy. To take care of us. To create this better world that we're dreaming of now. They tried simply to keep going. As we think about how we made it through, and how we'll keep making it through, and what recovery looks like, we owe it to them to remember how their actions carried us. We owe it to them, and to each other, to try something new.

When we think back to this time, we'll all have stories about how we coped. The bread we made, the puppies we brought home, the people we loved. We will have stories of how we connected and how we fell apart. And we'll have stories about the women in our own lives who kept us going—the women who didn't make headlines or books, but who checked in on us, who made us laugh, who were there when we cried. They made the isolation and the fear and the grief a little easier to bear. You know these women. They're your best friends, your neighbours, your partners, your mothers and grandmothers and sisters and aunts. They are your teachers and coaches. You *are* these women. You're the mom who hugged your shaking daughter after a nightmare about a world ending, who tried to remember integers and prime numbers and square roots, who worked hours into the night so your kids wouldn't be lonely in the sun. You're the friend who dropped off chocolate-stuffed care packages, who organized wine night on Zoom, who always picked up the phone. You're the one who volunteered your time, freely gave your support, did the best you could. You're the one who tried.

I know these women, too. At the beginning of the pandemic, I was invited to join a virtual card night with my aunt and two of her friends. We started with euchre, and when one week piled on into one month, then two, we switched to another game, at random, called 500—I'm not going to explain the rules, or the game itself, because I'm still not entirely sure what they are. We played one round after another, making mistakes and glorious gambles, always agreeing to "just one more," long past regular weeknight bedtimes, through yawns and bad plays and friendly taunts. We played to stay connected and grounded, and I'm not being hyperbolic when I say these women kept me sane. They were not the only ones. For months, my friends were there, unwavering, in group chats and on the phone. We were there for each other when loneliness and instability clawed at us, through lost jobs and struggling kids, through the anxieties of working from home and the anxieties of returning to work. We shared cat photos and photos of our newest sweatsuits, swapped recipes and face mask tips. We lifted each other up. We taught each other how to use Zoom. We tried socially distanced barbecues and felt the bitter-sweetness of reunion without touch, embrace, or even a simple high five.

For months, I spoke to my mother nearly every day from my home in Toronto. My sister, who's in her twenties and is intellectually disabled, lives with her in B.C. They'd gather on Zoom, always half out of the frame, a photo of my teenaged face and bad hair staring at me from the wall behind them. We would talk about the strangeness of the world, and my sister would gather new items for show and tell. She showed me the rock pets she made, decorated with colourful googly eyes and glitter paint that washed off in the valley mist, and I showed her my rock-like attempts at baking gluten-free bread, each batch rising slight centimetres higher. We rated her new scented Crayola markers, and even though I couldn't smell them, we both knew the pizza one was gross. I dragged my seventeen-year-old cat on camera, which he curmudgeonly allowed for brief seconds. My mom started making her own bath and beauty products during the quarantine, eventually customizing lavender-and-bergamot shampoo, lotion, face wash, and even perfume for me, which she'd send in hulking care packages. We celebrated Mother's Day, my sister's birthday, and my own birthday in this way, over Zoom, willing our love to seep through the screen, carried in sound waves and pixels.

Through all this love, we also helped each other bear loss. As some businesses and community centres opened, others didn't make it. For many heartbreaking weekends in a row, I helped tear down my historic boxing club. We sold all the equipment—the heavy bags and the speed bags and the weights and medicine balls—that helped me make it through the toughest times in my life. Piece by piece, we dismantled the place where I, and countless others, learned how to be strong. We categorized history into boxes and took it all to a storage locker, hoping, praying, vowing that one day we would take it all out again. We sat with our coach for hours, listening to her stories of how she built this special place, witnessing our grief, watching the biggest dragonfly we'd all ever seen flit through our increasingly empty gym and telling each other that, yes, it was a symbol of new beginnings. We cried. And, together, we gathered—the current crew of boxers and the many people who had, over the decades, also found something special in that special place—and we painted over our logo on the wall, returning it to its original state. Then, we rallied in the park to keep on training, masks on, socially distanced but connected, sweating in the blistering summer sun and then the cool fall breeze. There, we taught ourselves the meaning of resilience and community and strength all over again.

This book cannot capture the stories of every woman who's making a difference during the pandemic, of every woman who has suffered a loss. This pandemic is ongoing, and its effects will stretch further still. The tally, on both fronts, is ongoing.

This book also can't correct every history text that tells the story of human accomplishment and suffering through the eyes of men, too often reducing women to a footnote or an exception or nothing at all. It cannot recover those lost narratives, that particular grief. What I hope, though, is that this book has helped to capture an extraordinary moment in time, and the women who defined it. Their stories, their actions, and their voices matter. When we remember this time, and all that we have lost, we will not lose them, too. They were here. We were here.

Epilogue

Throughout the course of the pandemic, I've heard many variations of the same joke-but-not-a-joke: time is broken. There is so much happening, all at once, that every day feels like it's been stuffed with a whole year's worth of events—kind of like a pandemic olive. But also nothing is happening. What even are days of the week? Does it matter if it's a Tuesday or a Saturday? Days blend into each other, mixed by loneliness, exhaustion, isolation, loss. While writing *Women of the Pandemic*, I felt that time-bending keenly. Throughout the summer, as I interviewed dozens of women, it looked like Canada was flattening the curve. Empty streets filled. People appeared on patios, suddenly, as if by teleportation, laughing and drinking cold beers, chilled wine. We flocked to malls, gyms, weddings, potlucks, baseball diamonds, and soccer fields. With trepidation we planned for school, transforming classrooms and prepping remote learning. Public health measures softened, allowing openings and larger crowds. Our own rule-following slid, too. Maybe we were in denial, wrapped in dangerous conspiracies and twinning beliefs that the virus wouldn't touch us, that it wasn't that bad. Maybe we thought we were invincible. Maybe we simply missed our families, our friends, our regular lives.

Multiple infectious disease experts had told me that, in the entire history of pandemics, there had never been one that escaped the second wave. I knew this from researching disease across the centuries. The bubonic plague, cholera, the so-called Spanish flu, H1N1, SARS, and so on. Call it a wave or a phase or an unfortunate comeback, most disease outbreaks returned, ebbing and then crashing, seemingly disappearing and then reappearing elsewhere like a sneezing Houdini. Still, at one point this summer, I began to hope that by the time this book was published the pandemic would essentially be over in Canada. That wilfully naive hope bubbled into the fall, until reality popped it on September 28. That day, Ontario, my home province, recorded the highest number of new COVID-19 cases in a single day since the beginning of the pandemic, hitting seven hundred. It would go on to break that record a few days after that, and would break the new record a few days after that. On October 25, it reported more than one thousand cases in a single day. Around that time, Canada itself passed a grim milestone of two hundred thousand total cases, and our increasing daily count prompted the European Union to remove us from its "white list" of countries from which travellers can visit unrestricted. By the end of the month, the virus had killed over ten thousand people in Canada. People cancelled Thanksgiving plans, then Halloween trick-or-treating.

Winter holidays seemed up in the air, and even Trudeau suggested Christmas might be cancelled. And, of course, weeks later, it was.

As I write this, in the first days of 2021, nearing ten months into the pandemic, I can honestly say I have no idea what state the world will be in when *Women of the Pandemic* is published. By the time we rung in the new year, a total of about 85.1 million people, worldwide, had contracted the virus. Roughly 47.8 million of them had recovered, and 1.84 million of them had died. In Canada, cases among twentysomethings have surged, surpassing the number of cases of those in the eighty-plus age range near the end of August. A month before that, a globally focused study revealed that COVID-19 affected more middle-aged people than initially assumed. In England, it found, a person aged fifty-five to sixty-four "who gets infected with SARS-CoV-2 faces a fatality risk that is more than 200 times higher than the annual risk of dying in a fatal car accident." Meanwhile, back home, many provinces seemed hesitant to reinstate lockdown measures, and moved slowly. One day before Halloween, more than a dozen doctors in Manitoba published a letter urging the government to once more shut down the province. "We're well past the stage where even a robust community response will significantly slow the epidemic," they wrote in the *Winnipeg Free Press*. "Fortunately, your government has already shown us what needs to be done." Perhaps unfortunately, however, few seemed to want to do it all over again—even as many doctors warned of an overloaded system. Bonnie Henry advised a press conference at the end of October, "We are in the danger zone and we need to take the action to make it okay," but added that a renewed lockdown wouldn't be one of the measures.

By mid-November, Henry had changed her mind. On the nineteenth, the province entered a social lockdown, once again suspending events and social gatherings. Bars and restaurants were allowed to remain open (although not for New Year's Eve celebrations). A beleaguered Manitoba enacted even stricter measures that same month, largely closing everything but schools and daycare. Restaurants once more moved to take-out only, and retailers to online shopping and curbside pick-up. My home province, Ontario, waited longer to rewind time, first issuing a renewed and adjusted lockdown in hotspots, like Toronto, before eventually extending the orders province-wide on December 26. As emergency room doctor Kanna Vela said when I spoke to her again that month, the rising case counts that sparked all those closures had renewed the sense of fear for many frontline workers: "It's fear we won't beat this thing, fear more people will continue to die, fear we will run out of hospital beds and ventilators—something that is actually happening right now." She felt immense guilt, too, every day wondering if she'd bring the virus home to her family. But she also felt pride and obligation and a sense of privilege that, as the second wave crushed Canada, she was able to help many people who were at their most vulnerable.

After close to a year spent talking to essential workers and women on the front line, to those who've lost their livelihoods and their well-being, it was hard not to feel dismayed, and even a little angry, as I watched our case count steadily slope upwards in the final months of 2020. There is a reason the term *doomscrolling* seems so apt—we can't stop reading the news, even though we know it's depressing, disheartening, and just plain bad. I can see why some would want to turn away. I have, by now, spent months immersing myself in COVID-19 news, and the knowledge can be suffocating. No matter your vantage point, watching the pandemic unfold can often feel like riding a looping rollercoaster that's also screeching toward a cliff. The problem, of course, is that even if we safely parachute off the world's least fun ride, it's still going to crash over the edge. And there is a stark differ-ence between understandably shutting our eyes for a few moments and pretending there is nothing to be afraid of at all. Dampening the second wave is our collective govern-ments' responsibility, but let's face it, it's also ours.

If the end of 2020 saw overwhelming case counts and the terrifying emergence of a new, more contagious strain, it also saw hope. Canada approved and bought two vaccines in December, with the rollout beginning that same month. Still, as we know, that rollout is far from instantaneous—or easy. Each province and territory has planned out its own phases, deciding who gets their shot in the arm when. It's likely the general public won't all get their shots until the end of Sep-tember 2021, and that's if the rollout goes smoothly in each jurisdiction. Until then, we have another long slog ahead of us as we try to keep everyone safe from COVID-19.

Somewhere in the past, we were promised flying cars and jetpacks, and instead we got a pandemic that fractured the world. Many people have described 2020 as the worst year ever. I get it. I have, too. Unfortunately, the start of 2021 hasn't given us a blank slate. Even as we have a sense of renewed hope, the virus is still very much here and it can still feel like everything is out of our control. But that isn't entirely true: we can control how we move forward. We can control how we rebuild.

Memory is an unreliable thing. We can often erase or minimize problems with which we don't want to grapple. In this manner, we've allowed the measles and other preventable diseases to return. We were surprised at how strikingly similar the 1918 flu pandemic was to today's pandemic, both in its global sweep and in the way that strong public health measures had the ability to strike it down. When we recover from any illness, pandemic-wrought or not, we may even let our sense of how bad it was, how violently sick we were, fade. When the H1N1 pandemic struck, I was working as a reporter in Iqaluit, Nunavut, where people were especially hard-hit by the virus. I got it, too, and my cough became so chronic, and so vicious, that I eventually began to hack up blood—a side effect that lingered for weeks. I didn't think about it much in the intervening years. As for forgetting, you might think that's fairly harmless. But it can become dangerous in its own way.

Say, the way much of colonial Canada dismissed—and didn't learn from—the H1N1 pandemic because Indigenous, Northern, and remote communities bore the brunt of the outbreak. Or the ways in which too little change took place to prevent healthcare workers from getting sick, or suffering from the mental health fallout, post-SARS. How, on a wider scale, we didn't heed the many warnings from virologists and other experts that, if things didn't change, the next big pandemic would be a zoonotic one; that we should prepare for it. (As COVID-19 proved, many countries didn't.) These are the ways in which our dominant culture rewrites, or steamrolls over, other narratives. These are the ways in which we practise our own forgetting. It isn't always malicious, but it is usually unwise.

This book covers a moment in time—a small, but I think important, part of the pandemic. I wrote *Women of the Pandemic* because I believe it is essential that we remember these women and this point in history. Their bravery, their losses, their creativity, their activism, and their resilience will help lead us forward as we recover this year, and the next, and all the years after. We don't know what will happen to the world as we try to define a new normal. But we do know that, if we forget again, whatever we build next will be poorer for it. At the end of October, Theresa Tam released her annual report on the state of public health in Canada. Needless to say, it was unlike any annual health report before it. More than that, the report acknowledged, in writing, that we were not quite "all in it together"; many populations and groups suffered more than others. Tam also offered a new perspective on certain often-quoted statistics—for example, the fact that the overwhelming majority of those who were hospitalized, or died in hospital, had underlying conditions. Tam reframed the weird reassurance that only the previously unhealthy are at risk for what it was: a failure in the health system to care for those pre-existing conditions. Many of those people were sick because they were already at risk, doubly neglected.

The nod was refreshing. So too was the rest of the report, which stressed the interconnected nature of the pandemic and the necessarily interconnected nature of any proposed recovery plan. "The bottom line," she wrote in the report, is that "no one is protected until everyone is protected." It's a flip on the "we're all in it together" line, and one that feels not only more honest but more helpful. At a later press conference, Tam expanded on the sentiment, adding that she sees COVID-19 as a catalyst for collaboration among health, social, and economic sectors, as well as different levels of governance. She went on to echo something many of the women I interviewed also asked me: "Why can't we have those governance structures beyond the crisis and into recovery?" It's questions like this from those in power that give me hope for our future, in pandemic times and beyond.

Notes

Introduction

1 **Science was still unable to definitively explain:** World Health Organization, "Coronavirus disease 2019 (COVID-19) situation report –94," April 23, 2020, https://www.who.int/docs/default-source/coronaviruse /situation-reports/20200423-sitrep-94-covid-19.pdf?sfvrsn=b8304bf0_2; Smriti Mallpaty, "Animal source of the coronavirus continues to elude scientists," *Nature*, May 18, 2020, https://www.nature.com/articles /d41586-020-01449-8.

1 **including at least a dozen others who suddenly arrived in the city's hospitals:** Chaolin Huang, et al., "Clinical features of patients infected with 2019 novel coronavirus in Wuhan, China," *The Lancet* 395, no. 10223 (February 15, 2020): 497–506, https://www.thelancet.com/journals/lancet /article/PIIS0140-6736(20)30183-5/fulltext.

2 **In less than a week, the number of cases climbed from forty-one to fifty-nine:** Sui-Wee Lee and Donald G. McNeil Jr., "China identifies new virus causing pneumonialike illness," *New York Times*, January 8, 2020, https://www.nytimes.com/2020/01/08/health/china-pneumonia -outbreak-virus.html.

2 **By January 19, both the Chinese government and the World Health Organization (WHO) had estimated:** "Timeline of WHO's response to COVID-19," World Health Organization, September 9, 2020, https:// www.who.int/news-room/detail/29-06-2020-covidtimeline.

2 **Four days later, China abruptly closed Wuhan's borders:** Amy Qin and Vivian Wang, "Wuhan, center of coronavirus outbreak, is being cut off by Chinese authorities," *New York Times*, January 24, 2020, https://www .nytimes.com/2020/01/22/world/asia/china-coronavirus-travel.html.

3 **which has not been eradicated and which had, by the end of 2019, killed over 850 people:** "Middle East respiratory syndrome coronavirus (MERS CoV)," World Health Organization, https://www.who.int /emergencies/mers-cov/en/.

3 **"There are things that should frighten you about this coronavirus,"
she added:** Tristan Bronca, "The 2019 coronavirus is not like SARS,"
Canadian Healthcare Network, January 31, 2020, https://www
.canadianhealthcarenetwork.ca/the-2019-coronavirus-is-not-like-sars.

5 **In Canada, women comprise 81 per cent of healthcare workers:**
"Employment by class of worker, annual," Statistics Canada, https://
www150.statcan.gc.ca/t1/tbl1/en/cv.action?pid=1410002701.

5 **during nationwide shutdowns, and that racialized women, specifically,
held more essential jobs than anybody else:** Campbell Robertson and
Robert Gebelof, "How millions of women became the most essential
workers in America," *New York Times*, April 18, 2020, https://www
.nytimes.com/2020/04/18/us/coronavirus-women-essential-workers.html.

6 **Women between the ages of twenty-five and fifty-four, in particular:**
Matt Lundy, "Women, younger workers bear brunt of one million job
losses in March," *Globe and Mail*, April 9, 2020, https://www
.theglobeandmail.com/business/economy/article-canada-loses-record-1
-million-jobs-as-coronavirus-fallout-slams/.

6 **Economists began calling the chilling economic nosedive in North
America the "she-cession":** Erica Alini, "Welcome to the 'she-session.'
Why this recession is different," Global News, May 9, 2020, https://
globalnews.ca/news/6907589/canada-coronavirus-she-session/.

6 **as COVID-19 swept through long-term care (LTC) homes in Canada
at twice the rate:** Cassandra Szklarski, "Canada's proportion of
COVID-19 deaths in long-term care double the average of other
countries, study shows," CBC News, June 25, 2020, https://www.cbc.ca
/news/health/coronavirus-canada-long-term-care-deaths-
study-1.5626751; "CIHI snapshot: Pandemic experience in the long-term
care sector," Canadian Institute for Health Information, 2020, https://
www.cihi.ca/sites/default/files/document/covid-19-rapid-response-long
-term-care-snapshot-en.pdf?emktg_lang=en&emktg_order=1.

6 **only places in the world where more women than men:** Les Perreaux,
"Women make up over half of COVID-19 deaths in Canada, counter to
trends in most of world," *Globe and Mail*, May 21, 2020, https://www
.theglobeandmail.com/canada/article-women-make-up-over-half-of
-covid-19-deaths-in-canada-counter-to/.

8 **B.C.'s Henry, easily the most popular of the bunch, even got her own
fan club:** https://www.fluevog.com/shop/6155-dr-henry-pink-burgundy.

9 **In June, the *New York Times* ran a profile of her under the headline
"The Top Doctor Who Aced the Coronavirus Test":** Catherine Porter,
"The top doctor who aced the coronavirus test," *New York Times*, June 5,
2020, https://www.nytimes.com/2020/06/05/world/canada/bonnie
-henry-british-columbia-coronavirus.html.

9   **Trenches opened on New York's Hart Island, packed with unadorned wood boxes:** "In pictures: The novel coronavirus outbreak," CNN, November 19, 2020, https://www.cnn.com/2020/03/19/world/gallery /novel-coronavirus-outbreak/index.html.

9   **In Brooklyn, bodies in garish orange bags hemmed hospital hallways and loading bays:** Miriam Elder, "Nurse shared a harrowing photo of COVID-19 victims to show how horrifying the Outbreak is," Buzzfeed News, March 29, 2020, https://www.buzzfeednews.com/article/ miriamelder/coronavirus-new-york-city-hospital-nurse-covid-19-deaths; Jackie Salo, "Disturbing photos show body bags fill hallways of Brooklyn hospital amid coronavirus," *New York Post*, April 5, 2020, https://nypost .com/2020/04/05/disturbing-photos-show-body-bags-in-hallways-of -nyc-hospital-amid-coronavirus/.

14   **"By this point it's become clear that the pandemic is not the 'great equalizer'":** Yue Qian and Sylvia Fuller, "COVID-19 and the gender employment gap among parents of young children," University of Toronto Press Journals 46, no. S2 (August 2020): S89–S101, https://utpjournals .press/doi/pdf/10.3138/cpp.2020-077.

15   **Already we've seen a widening gender pay gap, an uneven return to work:** "COVID-19: A gender lens," UNFPA technical brief, March 2020, https://www.unfpa.org/sites/default/files/resource-pdf/COVID-19_A _Gender_Lens_Guidance_Note.pdf; Kendra Mangione, "When it comes to going back to work, COVID-19 is impacting Canadian mothers more than fathers: Study," CTV News, July 7, 2020, https://bc.ctvnews.ca /when-it-comes-to-going-back-to-work-covid-19-is-impacting-canadian -mothers-than-fathers-study-1.5014244?fbclid=IwAR2yHAcNN6B xOLVWzQxNsdKfzwYKA1z1YmQwFlZUcFUfluhwloCMefCChOg.

One: The Pandemic Arrives

17   **Every year, her team also screens returning travellers:** "Middle East respiratory syndrome coronavirus (MERS-CoV)," World Health Organization, https://www.who.int/emergencies/mers-cov/en/.

18   **A fifty-six-year-old man who had been travelling:** "First imported case of 2019 novel coronavirus in Canada, presenting as mild pneumonia," *The Lancet* 395 (February 13, 2020): 734, https://doi.org/10.1016/.

21   **Launched in 2008, PHO is a direct result, as the organization's first annual report puts it, of "Ontario's wake-up call from a series of outbreaks":** Public Health Ontario, Annual Report 2008–9, https://www .publichealthontario.ca/-/media/documents/a/2008/annual-report -2008-09.pdf?la=en.

21   **the province was in the midst of a listeriosis outbreak linked to contaminated cold cuts from Maple Leaf Foods:** "Report of the

independent investigator into the 2008 listeriosis outbreak," https://www
.canada.ca/en/news/archive/2009/07/report-independent-investigator
-into-2008-listeriosis-outbreak.html.

22   **About a week later, on Saturday, January 11, Chinese health authorities
     released the full sequence for SARS-CoV-2:** Institut Pasteur, "Whole
     genome of novel coronavirus, 2019-nCoV, sequenced," *ScienceDaily*,
     January 31, 2020, https://www.sciencedaily.com/releases/2020/01
     /200131114748.htm.

26   **the Program for Monitoring Emerging Diseases, or ProMED-mail, a
     free email service with over eighty thousand subscribers—the same
     service from which Allen received her January 3 alert:** ProMED,
     https://promedmail.org/about-promed/.

26   **The estimated case count was "apparently" twenty-seven:** ProMED,
     December 30, 2019, https://promedmail.org/promed-post/?id=6864153.

28   *January 23: 570. January 30: 7,818. January 31: 9,800*: Derrick Bryson
     Taylor, "A timeline of the coronavirus pandemic," *New York Times*,
     August 6, 2020, https://www.nytimes.com/article/coronavirus-timeline.
     html; https://www.who.int/docs/default-source/coronaviruse/situation
     -reports/20200130-sitrep-10-ncov.pdf?sfvrsn=d0b2e480_2.

30   **Not only was SARS-CoV-2 new, but science had only recognized the
     wider coronavirus family:** "Understanding SARS-CoV-2 and the drugs
     that might lessen its power," *The Economist*, March 12, 2020, https://www
     .economist.com/briefing/2020/03/12/understanding-sars-cov-2-and-the
     -drugs-that-might-lessen-its-power.

31   **Even then, when the close biological copy of SARS-CoV-2 struck,
     many virologists in Canada were still focused on other, more lethal
     things—Zika, West Nile, HIV:** Samira Mubareka, TheFutureEconomy,
     "Covid-19 research: Genomics, rapid execution & funding," April 27, 2020,
     https://thefutureeconomy.ca/interviews/samira-mubareka/.

31   **The coronavirus will then hijack the cell's machinery, creating endless
     doppelgangers:** Meredith Wadman, Jennifer Couzin-Frankel, Jocelyn
     Kaiser, and Catherine Matacic, "A rampage through the body," *Science*,
     April 24, 2020, https://science.sciencemag.org/content/368/6489
     /356?fbclid=IwAR2WoMUA4nImPFU5YNqkEibIj5QMFeWoxYdGu
     OxheLN1aUEZzXfqBncqSQc.

31   **Within their core, coronaviruses all have a strand of RNA, similar to
     DNA in that it contains the genetic information of the virus:** "What
     are the parts of a coronavirus?", Scripps.edu, https://www.scripps.edu
     /covid-19/faqs/parts-of-a-coronavirus/.

32   **In 1933, scientists isolated the influenza A virus using ferrets:**
     "Epidemiology and prevention of vaccine-preventable diseases: Influenza,"

https://www.cdc.gov/vaccines/pubs/pinkbook/flu.html; Claude Hannoun, "The evolving history of influenza viruses and influenza vaccines," *Expert Review of Vaccines* 12, no. 9 (2013): 1085–94, https://www.medscape.com/viewarticle/812621.

32 **Known as Vero cells, and first derived in 1962 from a dissected monkey in Japan:** "Cell line profile: Vero," Public Health England, https://www.phe-culturecollections.org.uk/media/122249/vero-cell-line -profile.pdf; Roxanne Khamsi, "Scientists may be using the wrong cells to study Covid-19," *Wired*, August 6, 2020, https://www.wired.com/story /scientists-may-be-using-the-wrong-cells-to-study-covid-19/.

33 **A human cell is about 10,000 nanometres; a coronavirus is 90 nanometres:** "Lesson 2: Scale of objects," NanoSense, https://nanosense .sri.com/activities/sizematters/sizeandscale/SM_Lesson2Student.pdf.

35 **The first worldwide case was reported in Mexico on March 18, 2009:** "2009 H1N1 Pandemic Resources," Infection Prevention and Control Canada, https://ipac-canada.org/pandemic-h1n1-resources.php.

36 **During the 1918 Spanish flu pandemic, mortality rates were particularly high for children under age five:** Centers for Disease Control and Prevention, "1918 pandemic (H1N1 virus), https://www.cdc.gov/flu /pandemic-resources/1918-pandemic-h1n1.html.

36 **Children also suffered more during swine flu:** Centers for Disease Control and Prevention, "2009 H1N1 pandemic (H1N1pdm09 virus)," https://www.cdc.gov/flu/pandemic-resources/2009-h1n1-pandemic.html.

38 **"This produced unnecessary delays and created confusion in populations who often were getting mixed messages":** Joshua Loomis, *Epidemics: The Impact of Germs and Their Power over Humanity* (Westport, CT: Praeger Publishers, 2018).

38 **"The challenge in all of this is it's unprecedented":** Sharon Kirkey, "Stopping Covid-19 could require eight months of 'aggressive social distancing,' outbreak modelling shows," *National Post*, March 21, 2020, https://nationalpost.com/health/could-the-covid-19-crisis-mean-well -be-social-distancing-for-eight-months-or-more.

39 **A century after that, a plague caused an under-attack Britain to seek help:** "Pandemics that changed history," April 1, 2020, History.com, https://www.history.com/topics/middle-ages/pandemics-timeline.

40 **By then, it had caused the deaths of some fifty million people:** "How pandemics change society," TheWeek.com, May 24, 2020, https:// theweek.com/articles/915738/how-pandemics-change-society; Elizabeth Kolbert, "Pandemics and the shape of human history," *The New Yorker*, April 6, 2020, https://www.newyorker.com/magazine/2020/04/06 /pandemics-and-the-shape-of-human-history.

40   **Smallpox, or the "speckled monster":** Christopher J. Rutty, "A pox on our history," CanadasHistory.ca, April 7, 2020, https://www.canadashistory.ca /explore/science-technology/a-pox-on-our-nation#:~:text=Smallpox %20began%20to%20shape%20Canada's,North%20American%20fur %2Dtrading%20post.

40   **both facilitated colonialism and decimated a way of life—likely deliberately:** Joshua Ostroff, "How a smallpox epidemic forged modern British Columbia," *Maclean's*, August 1, 2017, https://www.macleans.ca /news/canada/how-a-smallpox-epidemic-forged-modern-british -columbia/; Sarah Pruitt, "How colonization's death toll may have affected Earth's climate," History.com, January 31, 2019, https://www.history.com /news/climate-change-study-colonization-death-farming-collapse.

40   **It killed fifty million people and prevented the Americans from striking German reparations from the Treaty of Versailles, arguably paving the way for the Second World War:** "How pandemics change society," TheWeek.com, May 24, 2020, https://theweek.com/articles /915738/how-pandemics-change-society.

Two: Feeding a Country

50   **Stress-baking alone drove flour sales up 200 per cent:** "Canadian consumers adapt to Covid-19: A look at Canadian grocery sales up to April 11," Statistics Canada, May 11, 2020, https://www150.statcan.gc.ca /n1/pub/62f0014m/62f0014m2020005-eng.htm.

50   **These ambitious farmers ushered in an era of better treatment, a fledgling middle class, and a new economic model—a turning point now referred to as the birth of agrarian capitalism:** Adam McBride, "The Black Death led to the demise of feudalism. Could this pandemic have a similar effect?" Salon, April 26, 2020, https://www.salon.com /2020/04/26/the-black-death-led-to-the-demise-of-feudalism-could -this-pandemic-have-a-similar-effect/.

51   **As one union president put it, "Who in their right mind would risk contracting COVID . . . for $11.32 an hour?":** Steven Chase, "Grocery executives defend decision to cut $2-per hour 'hero' pay for workers," *Globe and Mail*, July 10, 2020, https://www.theglobeandmail.com /politics/article-grocery-executives-defend-decision-to-cut-covid-19 -pay-premiums-for/?utm_medium=Referrer:+Social+Network+ /+Media&utm_campaign=Shared+Web+Article+Links.

51   **in late March that such raises, along with other support programs, were "simply the right things to do":** Haley Ryan, "4 major Canadian grocers give front-line workers a raise during COVID-19 pandemic," CBC News, March 23, 2020, https://www.cbc.ca/news/canada/nova-scotia /sobeys-grocery-loblaw-metro-wages-pay-raise-covid-19-1.5506935.

52 **Then you'd hear about the Oshawa department manager who died:**
Bryan Passifiume, "Oshawa grocery store worker, 48, Ontario's youngest
COVID-19 death," CBC News, March 27, 2020, https://torontosun.com
/news/local-news/oshawa-grocery-store-worker-48-ontarios-youngest
-covid-19-death.

52 **the Vaughan distribution centre worker:** Bryann Aguilar, "Worker at
Ontario distribution plant dies after contracting COVID-19," CTV News,
May 8, 2020, https://toronto.ctvnews.ca/worker-at-ontario-distribution
-plant-dies-after-contracting-covid-19-1.4932054?cache=.

52 **the Walmart employee:** Tom Blackwell, "Hundreds infected, several
dead: How COVID-19 has affected the unsung essential workers in
retail," *National Post*, May 23, 2020, https://nationalpost.com/news
/canada/hundreds-infected-several-dead-how-covid-19-has-affected-the
-unsung-essential-workers-in-retail.

52 **"And by the time you get home, you've just got nothing in the tank":**
Perlita Stroh, "Stress, anxiety a heavy burden for people who can't work
from home or isolate properly," CBC News, May 12, 2020, https://www
.cbc.ca/news/health/covid-19-front-line-workers-stress-1.5561984.

52 **Loblaws, which said it had spent $180 million on extra wages,
clawed back wages first:** Susan Krashinsky Robertson, "Loblaws profit
falls as pandemic costs offset surging grocery revenue," *Globe and Mail*,
July 23, 2020, https://www.theglobeandmail.com/business/article
-loblaw-profit-falls-as-higher-costs-offset-grocery-revenue-surge/;
https://www.theglobeandmail.com/politics/article-grocery-executives
-defend-decision-to-cut-covid-19-pay-premiums-for/?utm_medium
=Referrer:+Social+Network+/+Media&utm_campaign=Shared+Web
+Article+Links.

53 **"We're being called essential workers," she said. "Well, you can't take
away essential":** "Scrapping $2 hourly bonus for grocery store workers
'a slap in the face': Loblaw baker," *As It Happens*, June 16, 2020, https://
www.cbc.ca/radio/asithappens/as-it-happens-tuesday-edition-1.5614169
/scrapping-2-hourly-bonus-for-grocery-store-workers-a-slap-in-the-face
-loblaw-baker-1.5614541.

53 **"That would be the right thing to do":** Steven Chase, "Grocery
executives defend decision to cut $2-per hour 'hero' pay for workers,"
Globe and Mail, July 10, 2020, https://www.theglobeandmail.com/
politics/article-grocery-executives-defend-decision-to-cut-covid-19
-pay-premiums-for/?utm_medium=Referrer:+Social+Network+
/+Media&utm_campaign=Shared+Web+Article+Links.

53 **In late August, eleven Loblaw-owned grocery stores in Newfoundland
went on strike:** "Loblaw-owned Dominion grocery store workers in N.L. on
strike over low wages, end of pandemic pay," *Globe and Mail*, August 23,

2020, https://www.theglobeandmail.com/business/article-loblaw
-owned-dominion-grocery-store-workers-in-nl-on-strike-over-low/.

53 **That same week, a Loblaws distribution centre in Surrey, B.C.,
announced a new outbreak:** Kathryn Tindale, "COVID-19 outbreak
at Surrey Loblaws warehouse, 80 new cases in B.C.," CityNews 1130,
August 20, 2020, https://www.citynews1130.com/2020/08/20/80
-cases-outbreak-at-loblaws/.

53 **A significant number of workers who briefly gained higher (but not
high) "hero" wages were women, many of them women of colour:**
Campbell Robertson and Robert Gebeloff, "How Millions of Women
Became the Most Essential Workers in America," *New York Times*, April 18,
2020, https://www.nytimes.com/2020/04/18/us/coronavirus-women
-essential-workers.html.

58 **She started to feel ill on Thursday, April 16, but finished her eight-
hour shift, sitting on cold metal as an:** https://www.facebook.com
/ActionDignity/; Licia Corbella, "Corbella: Cargill worker who died was
jolly, sweet and unprotected," *Calgary Herald*, May 5, 2020, https://
calgaryherald.com/opinion/corbella-cargill-worker-who-died-was-jolly
-sweet-and-unprotected.

58 **The day after that she was gone; Nguyen didn't even have a chance to
say goodbye:** Kathy Le, "'I am so, so sad': Grieving husband speaks out
after wife, a Cargill employee, succumbs to COVID-19," CTV News, May 4,
2020, https://calgary.ctvnews.ca/i-am-so-so-sad-grieving-husband-speaks
-out-after-wife-a-cargill-employee-succumbs-to-covid-19-1.4924500.

59 **Almost half of the plant's 2,000 workers had tested positive for
COVID-19:** Licia Corbella, "Corbella: Cargill worker who died was
jolly, sweet and unprotected," *Calgary Herald*, May 5, 2020, https://
calgaryherald.com/opinion/corbella-cargill-worker-who-died-was
-jolly-sweet-and-unprotected.

59 **The explanation for this disastrous record was both terrible and
simple:** Kathryn Blaze Baum, Carrie Tait, and Tavia Grant, "How Cargill
became the site of Canada's largest single outbreak of COVID-19," *Globe
and Mail*, May 2, 2020, https://www.theglobeandmail.com/business/
article-how-cargill-became-the-site-of-canadas-largest-single-outbreak-of/.

60 **Multiple employees told the *Globe* they were cleared to return despite
symptoms:** Kathryn Blaze Baum, Carrie Tait, and Tavia Grant, "How
Cargill became the site of Canada's largest single outbreak of COVID-19,"
Globe and Mail, May 2, 2020, https://www.theglobeandmail.com
/business/article-how-cargill-became-the-site-of-canadas-largest-single
-outbreak-of/.

60 **One *Calgary Herald* columnist described the announcement, thusly:
"It's a doozy filled with whoppers":** Licia Corbella, "Corbella: With

record COVID-19 outbreak Cargill's safety measures in question," *Calgary Herald*, April 30, 2020, https://calgaryherald.com/opinion/corbella-with-record-covid-19-outbreak-cargills-safety-measures-in-question/.

61 **"We put people first," it added:** "Statement on safety in Cargill's North American protein facilities," Cargill.com, July 15, 2020, https://www.cargill.com/story/statement-on-safety-in-cargill-north-american-protein-facilities.

61 **Combined with its other plant in Guelph, Ontario, Cargill has cornered more than 50 per cent of the beef processing market in Canada:** "Meat processing," Cargill.com, https://www.cargill.ca/en/meat-processing.

62 **"How are you making the most of the disruption?" one company update asked the workers:** Sara Mojtehedzadeh and Jennifer Yang, "More than 180 workers at this Toronto bakery got COVID-19—but the public wasn't informed. Why aren't we being told about workplace outbreaks?" *Toronto Star*, August 10, 2020, https://www.thestar.com/business/2020/08/10/more-than-180-workers-at-this-toronto-bakery-got-covid-19-but-the-public-wasnt-informed-why-arent-we-being-told-about-workplace-outbreaks.html?source=newsletter&utm_content=a01&utm_source=ts_nl&utm_medium=email&utm_email=3781EA08CD6F62E3775467109EAF689C&utm_campaign=lng_28933.

62 **By early June, more than 420 migrant farm workers had tested positive for COVID-19 across six operations in Ontario:** Tavia Grant and Kathryn Blaze Baum, "Migrant farm workers detail dangerous pandemic conditions," *Globe and Mail*, June 8, 2020, https://www.theglobeandmail.com/canada/article-farm-workers-detail-dangerous-pandemic-conditions/.

63 **Again, people reported testing positive for COVID but being told to keep working with others who'd also tested positive:** "Unheeded warnings: COVID-19 and migrant workers in Canada," Migrant Workers Alliance, June 2020, https://migrantworkersalliance.org/wp-content/uploads/2020/06/Unheeded-Warnings-COVID19-and-Migrant-Workers.pdf.

65 **Chilblains are caused by the inflammation of small blood vessels and can cause itching, swelling, blistering, and red or purple patches:** Roni Caryn Rabin, "What is 'covid toe'? Maybe a strange sign of Covid infection," *New York Times*, May 1, 2020, https://www.nytimes.com/2020/05/01/health/coronavirus-covid-toe.html.

65 **In the coming months, there would be considerable medical controversy over "COVID toes," with some studies denying the connection and others supporting it:** Wiley, "Study supports link between COVID-19

and 'COVID toes,'" *ScienceDaily*, July 2, 2020, https://www.sciencedaily
.com/releases/2020/07/200702113716.htm; Brooklyn Neustaeter, "New
study finds evidence between COVID-19 and 'COVID toes' symptom,"
CTV News, July 5, 2020, https://www.ctvnews.ca/health/coronavirus
/new-study-finds-evidence-between-covid-19-and-covid-toes-symptom
-1.5011460.

65   **In such cases, the SARS-CoV-2 virus was found in patients' sweat
glands:** C. Galván Casas, et al., "Classification of the cutaneous
manifestations of COVID-19: A rapid prospective nationwide consensus
study in Spain with 375 cases," *British Journal of Dermatology* 183, no. 1
(July 2020): 71–77, https://onlinelibrary.wiley.com/doi/full/10.1111
/bjd.19163; Wiley, "Study supports link between COVID-19 and 'COVID
toes,'" EurekAlert!, July 2, 2020, https://www.eurekalert.org/pub_releases
/2020-07/w-sslo70220.php.

Three: Communities Come Together

69   **Or, they'll pass the recently renovated St. Thomas United Baptist
Church:** Julian Abraham, "The Novascotian: Listen to the heartbeat of
North Preston," *Chronicle Herald*, April 9, 2020, https://www
.thechronicleherald.ca/lifestyles/local-lifestyles/the-novascotian-listen
-to-the-heartbeat-of-north-preston-435890/; Sherri Borden Colley,
"Newly renovated North Preston church reopens this weekend," CBC
News, September 7, 2017, https://www.cbc.ca/news/canada/nova-scotia
/fire-church-blacks-grand-reopening-pastor-st-thomas-united-baptist
-church-north-preston-1.4277615.

71   **As she and other community members watched the case counts climb
across the country:** Tim Bousquet, "Daily COVID-19 update: Possible
community spread case likely related to a St. Patrick's Day celebration
held in Lake Echo," *Halifax Examiner*, March 26, 2020, https://www
.halifaxexaminer.ca/province-house/daily-covid-19-update-possible
-community-spread-case-likely-related-to-a-st-patricks-day-celebration
-held-in-lake-echo/.

72   **As one community member would put it, "We don't get much help at
all. The little we do have, we have done it ourselves":** Robert Devet,
"Miranda Cain on COVID-19 and the Prestons: 'The little we do have,
we have done it ourselves.'" *Nova Scotia Advocate*, April 10, 2020, https://
nsadvocate.org/2020/04/10/miranda-cain-on-covid-19-and-the-prestons
-the-little-we-do-have-we-have-done-it-ourselves/.

73   **"And while we are using resources, doubling down on testing, and
trying to keep people healthy, the reckless and selfish few in these
communities are still having parties":** El Jones, "Daily COVID-19

update: Coronavirus hits the Black community, with a predictable racist response," *Halifax Examiner*, April 7, 2020, https://www.halifaxexaminer .ca/province-house/daily-covid-19-update-covid-19-hits-the-black -community-with-a-predictable-racist-response/; "Cape Breton woman in her 70s is Nova Scotia's first death related to COVID-19," CBC News, April 7, 2020, https://www.cbc.ca/news/canada/nova-scotia/covid-19 -death-nova-scotia-1.5524447.

73   **North Preston residents called out the premier's statements for what they were, and he refused to apologize:** Haley Ryan, "Preston group upset premier singled community out for COVID-19 criticism," CBC News, April 8, 2020, https://www.cbc.ca/news/canada/nova-scotia /preston-covid-19-premier-mcneil-nova-scotia-stigma-1.5526032.

73   **"And now we're fighting the battle of being from North Preston and Black and with an infectious disease":** Robert Devet, "Miranda Cain on COVID-19 and the Prestons: 'The little we do have, we have done it ourselves." *Nova Scotia Advocate*, April 10, 2020, https://nsadvocate.org /2020/04/10/miranda-cain-on-covid-19-and-the-prestons-the-little-we -do-have-we-have-done-it-ourselves/.

73   **Given the area's harsh history and continued maltreatment, many people understandably distrusted the system:** Emma Smith, "Preston community leaders work to get more people tested for COVID-19," CBC News, April 16, 2020, https://www.cbc.ca/news/canada/nova-scotia /east-preston-cherrybrook-preston-covid-19-response-team-testing -clinics-1.5534889.

74   **The release announcing the program said the cash would help people "put food on the table and keep a roof over their head":** "Canada Emergency Response Benefit to launch on April 6," Government of Canada, April 1, 2020, https://www.canada.ca/en/employment-social -development/news/2020/04/canada-emergency-response-benefit-to -launch-on-april-6.html.

74   **A group of Vancouver activists established a survival fund to dole out no-questions-asked increments of twenty-five to one hundred dollars:** https://www.gofundme.com/f/help-covid19-coming-together -vancouver?utm_medium=copy_link&utm_source=customer&utm _campaign=p_lico+share-sheet.

75   **An Indigenous artist named Lianne Spence raised funds to help buy and deliver groceries to elders in the Prince Rupert area:** Lee Wilson, "With her own work on hold, B.C. artist raises grocery money for elders during pandemic," APTN National News, April 8, 2020, https://www .aptnnews.ca/national-news/with-her-own-work-on-hold-b-c-artist -raises-grocery-money-for-elders-during-pandemic/.

76 **Two men had attacked a Toronto woman:** Dario Balca, "Toronto woman creates online network to help those vulnerable when travelling alone," CTV News, November 23, 2015, https://toronto.ctvnews.ca /toronto-woman-creates-online-network-to-help-those-vulnerable -when-travelling-alone-1.2671708.

78 **Justin Trudeau tweeted about the movement, saying, "We're only going to get through this by pulling together":** https://twitter.com /justintrudeau/status/1244820327051546630.

78 **Barack Obama called it "a great example of the kind of community spirit we need to get through this":** https://www.facebook.com /YMHECanada/photos/a-shout-out-to-all-the-canadian-caremongering -and-neighborhood-groups-organizing/1276260225904051/.

79 **In April, the** *Oxford English Dictionary*'s **senior editor called** *caremongering* **her favourite word to emerge from the pandemic:** Patricia Treble, "Tracking COVID-19's evolving language, from 'self-isolation' to 'social distancing,'" *Maclean's*, April 16, 2020, https:// www.macleans.ca/news/tracking-covid-19s-evolving-language-from -self-isolation-to-social-distancing/.

79 **The former pointed out that Canada is "a country whose inhabitants are stereotyped in the media as being kind to a fault":** Tom Gerken, "Coronavirus: Kind Canadians start 'caremongering' trend," BBC News, March 16, 2020, https://www.bbc.com/news/world-us-canada-51915723.

79 **The latter deemed caremongering "the antithesis in name and spirit to fearmongering":** David Moscrop, "In Canada, an inspiring movement emerges in response to the coronavirus," *Washington Post*, March 24, 2020, https://www.washingtonpost.com/opinions/2020/03/24/canada-an -inspiring-movement-emerges-response-coronavirus/.

79 **That realization, she said, came when a group in Malaysia helped three hundred stranded Rohingya refugees:** Erin Blakemore, "Who are the Rohingya people?" *National Geographic*, February 8, 2019, https://www .nationalgeographic.com/culture/people/reference/rohingya-people/.

79 **Though Human Rights Watch has condemned Malaysia's treatment of the thousands:** "Figures at a glance in Malaysia," UNHCR, https://www .unhcr.org/figures-at-a-glance-in-malaysia.html.

80 **"While there is an upside to this solidarity, it is often short-lived and romanticized by both media and politicians":** Yvonne Su, "The COVID-19 crisis has spawned a movement of helpers, but that doesn't relieve the government of its responsibility to protect the vulnerable," *Policy Options*, April 14, 2020, https://policyoptions.irpp.org/magazines /april-2020/caremongering-and-the-risk-of-happy-washing-during-a -pandemic/.

81 **For others, it made only slight or no impact:** Kate Allen, Jennifer Yang, Rachel Mendleson, and Andrew Bailey, "Lockdown worked for the rich, but not for the poor. The untold story of how COVID-19 spread across Toronto, in 7 graphics," *Toronto Star*, August 2, 2020, https://www.thestar.com/news/gta/2020/08/02/lockdown-worked-for-the-rich-but-not-for-the-poor-the-untold-story-of-how-covid-19-spread-across-toronto-in-7-graphics.html.

81 **Compared to the least diverse areas, the rate of hospitalization there was four times higher and the rate of death was twice as high:** Aaron Wherry, "One country, two pandemics: What COVID-19 reveals about inequality in Canada," CBC News, June 13, 2020, https://www.cbc.ca/news/politics/pandemic-covid-coronavirus-cerb-unemployment-1.5610404.

82 **In addition, Toronto discovered that newcomers and those living below the poverty line had higher case and hospitalization rates:** Ibid.

82 **Such dismal patterns were echoed in other cities:** Martin C. Barry, "Ongoing COVID-19 raises spectre of homelessness worsening," *Laval News*, August 25, 2020, https://www.lavalnews.ca/ongoing-covid-19-raises-spectre-of-homelessness-worsening/.

82 **When you're making sixty-two cents for every dollar a white man is paid, it's hard, if not impossible, to build an income cushion:** Erika Beras, "For Black women, the pay gap persists," Marketplace.org, August 13, 2020, https://www.marketplace.org/2020/08/13/pay-gap-black-womens-equal-pay-day/.

82 **To afford housing, many lower-income families also live together in smaller dwellings:** Aaron Wherry, "One country, two pandemics: What COVID-19 reveals about inequality in Canada," CBC News, June 13, 2020, https://www.cbc.ca/news/politics/pandemic-covid-coronavirus-cerb-unemployment-1.5610404; Leah Nairn, "The disproportionate impact of COVID-19 on Black women," COVID-19 Women's Initiative, June 5, 2020, https://covidwi.com/2020/06/05/the-disproportionate-impact-of-covid-19-on-black-women/.

83 **in May, one shelter went from handing out three or four hundred meals a week to well over six hundred:** Jennifer Ferreira, "The toll COVID-19 is taking on Canada's homeless," CTV News, May 22, 2020, https://www.ctvnews.ca/health/coronavirus/the-toll-covid-19-is-taking-on-canada-s-homeless-1.4950722.

83 **Plenty of them are also over sixty-five, the age at which COVID-19 health outcomes become more perilous, more grim:** Melissa Perri, Naheed Dosani, and Stephen H. Hwang, "COVID-19 and people experiencing homelessness: challenges and mitigation strategies," cmaj.ca, June 29, 2020, https://www.cmaj.ca/content/192/26/E716.

83   **All across the country, many of the services vulnerable populations relied on, including safe consumption sites, day programs, and food banks, were temporarily or permanently shuttered:** Jennifer Pagliaro, "City's busiest supervised injection site to reopen after month-long closure over COVID-19," *Toronto Star*, April 16, 2020, https://www.thestar.com/news/city_hall/2020/04/16/citys-busiest-supervised-injection-site-to-reopen-after-month-long-closure-over-covid-19.html; Alexandra Harvey, "Canadian food banks struggle to stay open, just as demand for their services skyrocket," *Globe and Mail*, April 11, 2020, https://www.theglobeandmail.com/canada/toronto/article-canadian-food-banks-struggle-to-stay-open-just-as-demand-for-their/.

83   **Fentanyl overdose deaths rose, and many shelters, including those who serve youth, reported being unable to access health care for those who were symptomatic:** Amanda Buchnea, Mary-Jane McKitterick, David French (2020). *Summary Report: Youth Homelessness and COVID-19: How the youth serving sector is coping with the crisis.* Toronto, ON: Canadian Observatory on Homelessness Press and A Way Home Canada, https://www.homelesshub.ca/sites/default/files/attachments/COVID-19_SUMMARY_REPORT%20%281%29_0.pdf; Amanda Coletta, "Canada's other health crisis: as overdoses surge, officials call on government to decriminalize illicit drugs," *Washington Post*, August 16, 2020, https://www.washingtonpost.com/world/the_americas/canada-drug-overdose-coronavirus/2020/08/15/559dabbe-dcd9-11ea-b4af-72895e22941d_story.html.

83   **In Toronto, a cluster of those hotels were located in the city's higher-income neighbourhoods; protestors rallied to denounce the "criminal element":** Muriel Draaisma, "Opposing groups demonstrate on same city street, to express views on midtown homeless shelters," CBC News, August 15, 2020, https://www.cbc.ca/news/canada/toronto/midtown-toronto-shelter-two-opposing-groups-protests-dual-rallies-1.5687994.

83   **In March, she was midway through a one-year fellowship sponsored by the Medical Psychiatry Alliance:** Hospital for Sick Children, "Psychiatry," http://www.sickkids.ca/psychiatry/CL-psychiatry-program/MPA/index.html.

87   **Talk of a repeat of the SARS outbreak, during which 43 per cent of those who caught the virus in Canada were healthcare workers, was already in the air:** Rima Styra, Laura Hawryluck, Susan Robinson, Sonja Kasapinovic, Calvin Fones, and Wayne L. Gold, "Impact on health care workers employed in high-risk areas during the Toronto SARS outbreak," January 24, 2008, https://www.ncbi.nlm.nih.gov/pmc/articles/PMC7094601/.

88   **They called themselves the Ontario COVID-19 Mental Health
      Network:** "About us," Ontario COVID-19 Mental Health Network,
      https://covid19therapists.com/about/; Rodolfo Rossi, et al., "Mental
      health outcomes among frontline and second-line health care workers
      during the Coronavirus Disease 2019 (COVID-19) pandemic in Italy,"
      JAMA Network Open, May 28, 2020, https://jamanetwork.com/journals
      /jamanetworkopen/fullarticle/2766378.

Four: Virus on the Front Line

100   **The nursing station itself sat in the blue, or "super clean" zone, which
      nobody could enter without washing their hands:** David W. Frost, et al.,
      "Principles for clinical care of patients with COVID-19 on medical units,"
      CMAJ 192, no. 26 (June 29, 2020), https://doi.org/10.1503/cmaj.200855.

103   **"Do you have a will?" she asked her staff, encouraging them to have an
      honest, compassionate conversation with their loved ones. "Powers of
      attorney for finance and personal care? Are all your insurance policies
      and financial documents organized and easy to find?":** Robyn Doolittle,
      Erin Anderssen, and Les Perreaux, "In Canada's coronavirus fight, front-line
      workers miss their families, fear the worst and hope they're ready," *Globe
      and Mail*, April 4, 2020, https://www.theglobeandmail.com/canada/
      article-in-canadas-coronavirus-fight-front-line-workers-miss-their-families.

105   **In fact, across the system, immigrants play a vital role in Canadian
      health care, accounting for one out of four workers:** Ranjit Bhaskar,
      "Looking Ahead: What Immigrant Health Workers on the Frontlines
      Mean for Canada," *New Canadian Media*, September 4, 2020, https://
      newcanadianmedia.ca/looking-ahead-what-immigrant-health-workers
      -on-the-front-lines-mean-for-canada.

106   **The vast majority of them were workers like Mojica: non-medical staff
      who showed up every day for their shifts, many of them because they
      couldn't afford not to:** Lauren Pelley, "Nurses, lab workers, physicians,
      among 'alarming' number of health-care workers with COVID-19," CBC
      News, May 15, 2020, https://www.cbc.ca/news/canada/toronto/health
      -care-workers-covid-19-alarming-rate-1.5568711.

106   **The first healthcare worker who died in the province was a hospital
      cleaner:** Chris Herhalt and Bryann Aguilar, "Brampton hospital cleaner
      becomes first Ontario health-care worker to die of COVID-19," CTV News,
      April 16, 2020, https://toronto.ctvnews.ca/brampton-hospital-cleaner
      -becomes-first-ont-health-care-worker-to-die-of-covid-19-1.4890298
      ?cache=%2F5-things-to-know-for-friday-november-15-2019-1.4687011.

107   **More alarmingly, it also showed that:** Long H. Nguyen, et al., "Risk of
      COVID-19 among front-line health-care workers and the general

community: A prospective cohort study," *Lancet Public Health* 5 (July 31, 2020): e475–83, https://www.thelancet.com/action/showPdf?pii=S2468 -2667%2820%2930164-X.

107 **In August, it estimated 62 percent of the healthcare workers it catalogued were people of colour:** Christina Jewett, "Health care workers of color nearly twice as likely as whites to get COVID-19," *The Guardian*, August 6, 2020, https://khn.org/news/health-care-workers -of-color-nearly-twice-as-likely-as-whites-to-get-covid-19.

108 **Another 43 per cent said they had faced threats or intimidation:** Maryam Shah, "Canadians of Chinese ethnicity report widespread racism over coronavirus: Survey," Global News, June 22, 2020, https:// globalnews.ca/news/7091118/coronavirus-racism-chinese-canadians; Ryan Flanagan, "StatCan survey shows new evidence of increase in anti-Asian sentiment, attacks," CTV News, July 9, 2020, https://www .ctvnews.ca/canada/statcan-survey-shows-new-evidence-of-increase-in -anti-asian-sentiment-attacks-1.5016027.

110 **The WHO reported that the share of true asymptomatic cases ranged anywhere from 6 to 41 per cent:** "Transmissions of SARS-CoV-2: Implications for infection prevention precautions," World Health Organ-ization, July 9, 2020, https://www.who.int/news-room/commentaries /detail/transmission-of-sars-cov-2-implications-for-infection-prevention -precautions.

110 **The U.S. Centers for Disease Control and Prevention (CDC) has estimated that 40 per cent of SARS-CoV-2 transmission has happened before people even feel ill:** Jacqueline Howard, "WHO clarifies comments on asymptomatic spread of coronavirus: 'There is much unknown,'" CTV News, June 9, 2020, https://www.ctvnews.ca/health/coronavirus /who-clarifies-comments-on-asymptomatic-spread-of-coronavirus -there-s-much-unknown-1.4976424.

118 **"It can attack almost anything in the body with devastating conse-quences," said one U.S.-based doctor that month. "Its ferocity is breathtaking and humbling":** Meredith Wadman, "A rampage through the body," *Science* 368, no. 6489 (April 24, 2020): 356–360, https:// science.sciencemag.org/content/368/6489/356?fbclid=IwAR2WoMUA 4nImPFU5YNqkEibIj5QMFeWoxYdGuOxheLN1aUEZzXfqBncqSQc.

118 **A subsequent research paper published in the *Lancet* termed the stages of infection as "the four horsemen of a viral apocalypse":** Pere Domingo, et al., "The four horsemen of a viral Apocalypse: The pathogenesis of SARS-CoV-2 infection (COVID-19)," *EBioMedicine* 58 (July 29, 2020), https://doi.org/10.1016/j.ebiom.2020.102887.

119 **An estimated 80 per cent of those infected with the virus remain asymptomatic, or only develop minor or moderate illness:** Ibid.

120 **At its deadliest, the virus seems insatiable, overtaking every part of the body it can:** Ross W. Paterson, et al., "The emerging spectrum of COVID-19 neurology: Clinical, radiological and laboratory findings," *Brain* 143, no. 10 (October 2020): 3104–3120, https://doi.org/10.1093/brain/awaa240; Apoorva Mandavilli, "How the coronavirus attacks the brain," *New York Times*, September 9, 2020, https://www.nytimes.com/2020/09/09/health/coronavirus-brain.html?action=click&module=Well&pgtype=Homepage&section=Health.

120 **Some studies have suggested that pre-existing conditions, like asthma and diabetes:** Lei Fang, George Karakiulakis, and Michael Roth, "Are patents with hypertension and diabetes mellitus at increased risk for COVID-19 infection?" *The Lancet* 8 (March 11, 2020), https://www.thelancet.com/action/showPdf?pii=S2213-2600%2820%2930116-8.

120 **the size of the initial viral load:** Elisabet Pujadas, "SARS-CoV-2 viral load predicts COVID-19 mortality," *The Lancet* 8 (August 6, 2020), https://doi.org/10.1016/ S2213-2600(20)30354-4.

121 **Considered to be the next level of therapy for COVID-19 when everything, even a ventilator, has failed, an ECMO machine:** Melissa Bailey, "Miracle machine makes heroic rescues—and leaves patients in limbo," Kaiser Health Network, June 18, 2020, https://khn.org/news/miracle-machine-makes-heroic-rescues-and-leaves-patients-in-limbo; Chris Herhalt, "Toronto hospital employs tool of last resort to save sickest COVID-19 patients," CP24, May 12, 2020, https://www.cp24.com/news/toronto-hospital-employs-tool-of-last-resort-to-save-sickest-covid-19-patients-1.4936197.

122 **"I went on autopilot":** May Warren, "Toronto Western hospital temporarily closes Covid ward to new patients as it tries to contain outbreak," *Toronto Star*, October 26, 2020, https://www.thestar.com/news/gta/2020/10/26/toronto-western-hospital-temporarily-closes-covid-ward-to-new-patients-as-it-tries-to-contain-outbreak.html.

124 **"COVID-19 is not a terrorist or intergalactic villain," wrote one healthcare worker. "Heroes are not necessary to kill a virus. Heroes are a symptom that our system has failed":** Daniel Barron, "Health care workers don't want to be heroes," *Scientific American*, June 21, 2020, https://www.scientificamerican.com/article/health-care-workers-dont-want-to-be-heroes.

Five: Crisis at Home

132 **Mothers also, perhaps unsurprisingly, did about two hours more housework every day:** Alison Andrew, et al., "Parents, especially mothers, paying heavy price for lockdown," Institute for Fiscal Studies, May 27, 2020, https://www.ifs.org.uk/publications/14861.

133 "The average length of an uninterrupted stretch of work time was three minutes, 24 seconds. The longest uninterrupted period was 19 minutes, 35 seconds. The shortest was mere seconds": "Yes, balancing work and parenting is impossible. Here's the data," *Washington Post*, https://www .washingtonpost.com/outlook/interruptions-parenting-pandemic-work -home/2020/07/09/599032e6-b4ca-11ea-aca5-ebb63d27e1ff_story .html?utm_campaign=wp_todays_headlines&utm_medium=email&utm _source=newsletter&wpisrc=nl_headlines&fbclid=IwAR3IExImHNhy2a WOtnf-gbGgg1_Z3cG7B3Foc8eJCowUzl9506-6_sjge7w.

135 **It was the first time she'd left her house since the lockdown had begun weeks earlier:** Andrea O'Reilly, "'Trying to function in the unfunctionable': Mothers and COVID-19," *Journal of the Motherhood Initiative* 11, no. 1 (2020), https://jarm.journals.yorku.ca/index.php /jarm/article/view/40588.

136 **"Why is nobody talking about how unsustainable this is for working parents?":** Claire Gagne, "Why is no one talking about how unsustainable this is for working parents?" *Today's Parent*, April 24, 2020, https://www .todaysparent.com/blogs/opinion/why-is-no-one-talking-about-how -unsustainable-this-is-for-working-parents.

136 **Some media cautioned of a "patriarchal pandemic":** Soraya Chemaly, "Coronavirus could hurt women the most. Here's how to prevent a patriarchal pandemic," NBC News, April 20, 2020, https://www .nbcnews.com/think/opinion/coronavirus-could-hurt-women-most-here -s-how-prevent-patriarchal-ncna1186581.

137 *The Atlantic* **got it right when it stated:** Helen Lewis, "The coronavirus is a disaster for feminism," *The Atlantic*, March 19, 2020, https://www .theatlantic.com/international/archive/2020/03/feminism-womens -rights-coronavirus-covid19/608302.

137 **In June, the *New York Times* warned again that:** Patricia Cohen and Tiffany Hsu, "Pandemic could scar a generation of working mothers," *New York Times*, June 3, 2020, https://www.nytimes.com/2020/06/03 /business/economy/coronavirus-working-women.html.

137 **"The consensus is that everyone agrees this is a catastrophe, but we are too bone-tired to raise our voices above a groan, let alone scream through a megaphone," she wrote:** Deb Perelman, "In the Covid-19 economy, you can have a kid or a job. You can't have both," *New York Times*, July 2, 2020, https://www.nytimes.com/2020/07/02/business /covid-economy-parents-kids-career-homeschooling.html.

137 **San Diego woman who'd been fired from her job because her boss could hear her young kids in the background on video calls:** Nicole Pelletiere, "Mom alleges in lawsuit she was fired for not keeping kids

quiet while working from home," *Good Morning America,* July 2, 2020, https://www.goodmorningamerica.com/family/story/mom-alleges -lawsuit-fired-keeping-kids-quiet-working-71574603.

138 **In the U.K., suspected domestic homicides tripled during the first month of lockdown:** Amanda Taub and Jane Bradley, "As domestic abuse rises, U.K. failings leave victims in peril," *New York Times,* July 2, 2020, https://www.nytimes.com/interactive/2020/07/02/world/europe /uk-coronavirus-domestic-abuse.html.

138 **"Since then, calls to our crisis line have increased by up to 300 per cent":** Meera Bains, "Battered Women Support Services asks for more volunteers amid COVID-19 pandemic," CBC News, August 29, 2020, https://www.cbc.ca/news/canada/british-columbia/battered-women -support-services-asks-for-more-volunteers-amid-covid-19-pandemic -1.5704691.

139 **If that damage did occur, the baby could develop congenital Zika syndrome, which has five key markers, including brain damage:** "Zika virus: Pregnant or planning a pregnancy," Government of Canada, https://www.canada.ca/en/public-health/services/diseases/zika-virus /pregnant-planning-pregnancy.html.

139 **It's worth noting that, six months into the pandemic:** Meredith Wadman, "Why pregnant women face special risks from COVID-19," *Science,* August 4, 2020, https://www.sciencemag.org/news/2020/08 /why-pregnant-women-face-special-risks-covid-19; Christina Caron, "Why we still don't know enough about COVID-19 and pregnancy," *New York Times,* July 10, 2020, https://www.nytimes.com/2020/07/10 /parenting/pregnancy/pregnancy-coronavirus-data.html.

Six: The She-cession

156 **On average, each business added $135,000 to its debt, with business owners relying on personal savings, credit cards, bank loans, and retirement savings (in that order):** "Debt knell: Small business COVID-19 debt totals $117 billion," Canadian Federation of Independent Business, July 15, 2020, https://www.newswire.ca/news-releases/debt -knell-small-business-covid-19-debt-totals-117-billion-827855593.html.

156 **By mid-September, only 18 per cent of businesses in Alberta were at or above normal revenues, though 65 per cent of them had reopened:** "Small business recovery dashboard," Canadian Federation of Independent Business, November 3, 2020, https://www.smallbusinesseveryday.ca /dashboard.

157 **In fact, in recognition of this, Justin Trudeau announced a $221 million funding program in September 2020:** "Prime Minister

announces support for Black entrepreneurs and business owners,"
Cision, September 9, 2020, https://www.newswire.ca/news-releases
/prime-minister-announces-support-for-black-entrepreneurs-and
-business-owners-869166674.html.

160 **Their province hadn't yet announced a state of emergency:** John Paul
Tasker, "The 'measure of last resort': What is the Emergencies Act and
what does it do?" CBC News, March 23, 2020, https://www.cbc.ca/news
/politics/trudeau-emergencies-act-premier-1.5507205.

162 **By October, more than 750,000 businesses had received CEBA loans,
totalling $30.24 billion:** "Canada Emergency Business Account (CEBA),"
Government of Canada, https://ceba-cuec.ca.

163 **The 2016 census shows that visible minorities comprise less than 10
per cent of Fredericton's population:** "Census profile, 2016 census,"
Statistics Canada, https://www12.statcan.gc.ca/census-recensement
/2016/dp-pd/prof/details/page.cfm?Lang=E&Geo1=POPC&Code1=0305
&Geo2=PR&Code2=13&SearchText=Fredericton&SearchType=Begins
&SearchPR=01&B1=All&GeoLevel=PR&GeoCode=0305&TABID=1
&type=0.

166 **And more than one-third modified their products or services—
compared to just over one-quarter of all businesses in Canada:** Jessica
Bossé, Shivani Sood, and Chris Johnston, "Impact of COVID-19 on
businesses majority-owned by women," Statistics Canada, July 17, 2020,
https://www150.statcan.gc.ca/n1/pub/45-28-0001/2020001/article
/00056-eng.htm.

166 **The closure curtailed several decades' worth of plans to sell the
restaurant:** Alexsandra Sagan, "Pandemic-related restaurant closures
take an emotional and financial toll," CBC News, June 1, 2020, https://
www.cbc.ca/news/business/restaurant-closures-covid-19-1.5592946.

166 **By the end of June, about 40 per cent of women-owned businesses
were forced to lay off employees:** "Staffing actions taken by businesses
during the COVID-19 pandemic, by business characteristics," Statistics
Canada, https://www150.statcan.gc.ca/t1/tbl1/en/tv.action?pid=3310023101.

166 **What's more, nearly two-thirds of those who did lay off workers sent
pink slips to 80 per cent of their staff:** Wendy Cukier, "COVID-19 may
turn back the clock on women's entrepreneurship," *The Conversation*,
June 29, 2020, https://theconversation.com/covid-19-may-turn-back
-the-clock-on-womens-entrepreneurship-139961.

167 **On top of that, small and medium-sized enterprises with under
twenty employees—the type of business women are more likely to
own—suffered disproportionately more revenue loss than larger
companies with over one hundred employees:** Jessica Bossé, Shivani

Sood, and Chris Johnston, "Impact of COVID-19 on businesses majority-owned by women," Statistics Canada, July 17, 2020, https://www150 .statcan.gc.ca/n1/pub/45-28-0001/2020001/article/00056-eng.htm.

167 **More women business owners reported being unable to pay their rent or mortgage payments:** Ibid.

168 **A full 80 per cent of racialized founders of all genders reported lost contracts, customers, or clients:** "Falling through the cracks," Canadian Women's Chamber of Commerce, May 2020, https://canwcc.ca/wp -content/uploads/2020/05/Falling-through-the-Cracks_CanWCC _May2020v19.pdf.

169 **All told, the pandemic plummeted women's participation in the labour force to 55 per cent, its lowest point in three decades:**"Pandemic threatens decades of women's labour force gains," *RBC Economics*, July 16, 2020, https://thoughtleadership.rbc.com/pandemic-threatens -decades-of-womens-labour-force-gains.

169 **In the first two months alone, 1.5 million women lost their jobs, sparking the term "she-cession":** Erica Alini, "Welcome to the 'she-session.' Why this recession is different," Global News, May 9, 2020, https:// globalnews.ca/news/6907589/canada-coronavirus-she-session.

169 **Women in the core working ages, between twenty-five and fifty-four, lost more than twice the number of jobs lost by men in the same age range:** Matt Lundy, "Women, younger workers bear brunt of one million job losses in March," *Globe and Mail*, April 9, 2020, https://www .theglobeandmail.com/business/economy/article-canada-loses-record-1 -million-jobs-as-coronavirus-fallout-slams.

170 **By the end of March, the government had 2.2 million EI claims on its virtual desk:** Jordan Press, "Behind the scenes: How CERB went from an idea to a reality," CTV News, May 3, 2020, https://www.ctvnews.ca /health/coronavirus/behind-the-scenes-how-cerb-went-from-an-idea -to-a-reality-1.4922682.

170 **One man reported making 1,700 phone calls before he got through, while others enlisted friends' and partners' phones to call from multiple numbers at once:** Karina Roman, "EI claimants are going weeks without income as federal call system slows to a crawl," CBC News, May 1, 2020, https://www.cbc.ca/news/politics/employment-insurance-ei-cerb -covid-coronavirus-pandemic-1.5549617.

170 **In the end, about 7,000 people raised their hands to step outside their regular jobs and help answer calls:** Samantha Beattie, "CERB call centre volunteer applauds kindness of Canadians during pandemic," *Huffington Post*, April 9, 2020, https://www.huffingtonpost.ca/entry/cerb-call -centre-canadian-kindness_ca_5e8f7ffdc5b6d641a6bbf0f7.

170   Or, as one woman put it in mid-April, "Finally got put on hold for
three hours . . . made two loaves of banana bread and at 4:35 p.m. they
answered. I swear I cried": David Molko, "Confused about applying for the
CERB? You're not alone," CTV News, April 21, 2020, https://bc.ctvnews.ca
/confused-about-applying-for-the-cerb-you-re-not-alone-1.4906340.

171   Many of them had stayed on CERB for months, holding tight to the
lifeline: "Canada Emergency Response Benefit statistics," Government
of Canada, https://www.canada.ca/en/services/benefits/ei/claims-report
.html.

171   Without her partner's help, she would have been in a "scary situation"
unable to buy food or pay her bills. "Sadly," she acknowledged, "I'm not
the only one in this situation": Meredith MacLeod, "Stories of CERB:
Canadians share how they're using the emergency benefit," CTV News,
June 17, 2020, https://www.ctvnews.ca/health/coronavirus/stories-of-cerb
-canadians-share-how-they-re-using-the-emergency-benefit-1.4931779.

172   He didn't (quite), but all the speculation only forced UBI more into
the mainstream conversation, something that was, largely, previously
unthinkable: Patrick Brethour, "With new benefits plan, Liberals move
toward guaranteed basic income," Globe and Mail, September 1, 2020,
https://www.theglobeandmail.com/business/article-liberals-revised
-covid-19-emergency-benefits-resemble-a-national.

172   "Yes, the government stepped up and helped but what that made me
realize is that this happens to families all the time": Nathan Martin,
"Edmontonians rally for universal basic income at legislature," Edmonton
Journal, September 19, 2020, https://edmontonjournal.com/news/local
-news/edmontonians-rally-for-universal-basic-income-at-legislature.

173   Compare that to construction or manufacturing, which, by fall 2020,
were looking at significantly shorter recovery timelines: "Small
business recovery dashboard," Canadian Federation of Independent
Business, November 3, 2020, https://www.smallbusinesseveryday.ca
/dashboard.

173   As one woman said in May, "Do I find a job first? Do I find child care?
How do I do one without the other?": "Without more support for child
care, economic recovery will be slow, says expert," The Current, May 22,
2020, https://www.cbc.ca/radio/thecurrent/the-current-for-may-22
-2020-1.5580159/without-more-support-for-child-care-economic-recovery
-will-be-slow-says-expert-1.5581464.

174   Already in April, Ontario landlords, for example, had reported a
10 per cent delinquency rate: Alastair Sharp, "Toronto renters in for a
'bloodbath' of evictions after pandemic ends, advocate warns," Toronto
Star, May 22, 2020, https://www.thestar.com/news/canada/2020/05

/22/toronto-renters-in-for-terrifying-bloodbath-of-evictions-after
-pandemic-ends.html.

174 **around the same time, about 760,000 Canadians had deferred
mortgage payments**: "Residential mortgage industry report," Canada
Mortgage and Housing Corporation, September 2020, https://assets
.cmhc-schl.gc.ca/sites/cmhc/data-research/publications-reports
/residential-mortgage-industry-report/2020/residential-mortgage
-industry-report-2020-en.pdf?rev=440a31e2-687a-43bf-a875-093e8f9b17d5.

Seven: Every Decision Counts

186 **She talked about how she was isolating herself from her family and
about the configuration of her house**: Dr. Deena Hinshaw, "Update on
COVID-19 – March 16, 2020," YourAlberta, streamed live on March 16,
2020, YouTube video, https://www.youtube.com/watch?v=5Tq1KgRwUDk
&list=PLvrD8tiHIX1L5LKwBokl-4aJjkK4OuE-l&index=97.

187 **One comment in particular seemed to sum it all up: "I know
everyone's asking, but are these for sale?"**: Erica O. (@_thegoodseed),
2020. Twitter, March 19, 2020, https://twitter.com/dinnerwithjulie/status
/1240760952502366208.

189 **They defied hate, deliberate misinformation, partisanship. Tam
openly, repeatedly condemned anti-Asian racism**: Kathleen Harris,
"Canada's chief public health officer condemns racist acts linked to
coronavirus outbreaks," CBC News, February 3, 2020, https://www.cbc.ca
/news/politics/tam-public-health-coronavirus-racism-1.5445713.

189 **(Whereas some male leaders, such as Ontario Conservative MP
David Sloan, who asked "Does [Tam] work for China?" and tweeted
"Dr. Tam must go! Canada must remain sovereign over decisions,"
instead focused on sowing division)**: Kathleen Harris, "Conservatives
blast MP who asked whether top pandemic doctor, 'works for China' as
Scheer steers clear," CBC News, April 23, 2020, https://www.cbc.ca/news
/politics/sloan-tam-china-coronavirus-pandemic-1.5542497.

191 **At the international level, studies of the world's 194 countries have
shown that women national leaders fared better in terms of both
infection and mortality rates**: Orla Barry, "It's official: Women are
better leaders in a pandemic," *The World*, August 31, 2020, https://
www.pri.org/stories/2020-08-31/its-official-women-are-better-leaders
-pandemic.

191 **As the *Guardian* put it, "Plenty of countries with male leaders . . .
have done well. But few with female leaders have done badly"**: Jon
Henley and Eleanor Ainge Roy, "Are female leaders more successful at
managing the coronavirus crisis?" *The Guardian,* April 25, 2020, https://

www.theguardian.com/world/2020/apr/25/why-do-female-leaders
-seem-to-be-more-successful-at-managing-the-coronavirus-crisis#.

191   **In April, the *Atlantic* even posited that Ardern may be "the most effective leader on the planet" for the way she was handling the pandemic**: Uri Friedman, "New Zealand's prime minister may be the most effective leader on the planet," *The Atlantic*, April 19, 2020, https://www.theatlantic.com/politics/archive/2020/04/jacinda-ardern-new -zealand-leadership-coronavirus/610237.

191   **As Ardern herself said when she announced increased mass shutdowns in her country, "The worst-case scenario is simply intolerable"**: Jacinda Ardern, "COVID-19 alert level increased," Beehive.govt.nz, March 23, 2020, https://www.beehive.govt.nz/speech/prime-minister -covid-19-alert-level-increased.

192   **Some of the N.W.T.'s thirty-three communities are home to only about a hundred people; one, Kakisa, has fewer than fifty residents**: "NWT Lifestyle," Government of the Northwest Territories, https://www.gov.nt.ca /careers/en/nwt-lifestyle.

192   **The community's chief, Dana Tizya-Tramm, politely told them to get lost**: Dirk Meissner, "Quebec couple who fled to remote Indigenous community to avoid COVID-19 sent back: Chief," Global News, March 31, 2020, https://globalnews.ca/news/6758430/coronavirus-quebec -couple-indigenous-yukon.

193   **By 2008, the TB rate among Indigenous people was six times higher than the overall Canadian rate**: "TB and Aboriginal people," Canadian Public Health Association, https://www.cpha.ca/tb-and-aboriginal-people.

193   **And while tuberculosis provides one of the starkest examples, it's well documented that Indigenous peoples across Canada experience higher rates**: J. Reading Ph.D., "The crisis of chronic disease among Aboriginal peoples: A challenge for public health, population health and social policy," University of Victoria Centre for Aboriginal Health Research, https://dspace.library.uvic.ca/bitstream/handle/1828/5380 /Chronic-Disease-2009.pdf?sequence=1&isAllowed=y.

193   **Those living in First Nation communities were 2.8 times more likely to be hospitalized from the flu strain, and had an ICU admission rate that was three times higher than that of non-Indigenous people**: Katya L. Richardson, Michelle S. Driedger, Nick J. Pizzi, Jianhong Wu, and Seyed M. Moghadas, "Indigenous populations health protection: A Canadian perspective," *BMC Public Health* (December 20, 2012), doi.org /10.1186/1471-2458-12-1098.

193   **Or, put another way: while Indigenous people represent only 4.3 per cent of the population, during the first wave of H1N1 they accounted**

for 27.8 per cent of hospitalizations and made up 25.6 per cent of critically ill patients in ICUs across Canada: "The 2009 H1N1 influenza pandemic among First Nations, Inuit and Métis peoples in Canada: Epidemiology and gaps in knowledge," National Collaborating Centres for Public/Aboriginal Health (2009), https://www.ccnsa-nccah.ca/docs /other/FS-InfluenzaEpidemiology-EN.pdf.

195   **Over the next few weeks, another four people tested positive in the territory:** "COVID-19 in NWT," Government of the Northwest Territories, https://www.gov.nt.ca/covid-19.

195   **The last of them recovered without incident in mid-April, and nobody else tested positive for months:** John Last, "No active cases of COVID-19 in N.W.T. as final patient recovers," CBC News, April 20, 2020, https://www.cbc.ca/news/canada/north/covid-19-nwt-all-cases -recovered-april-1.5538548.193 **In a way, it was almost familiar, too: during H1N1, Kandola had missed her youngest son's first birthday; she's missed a lot of stuff this time around, as well:** Danielle D'Entremont, "Meet the woman leading the territory with all COVID-19 cases resolved," CBC News, April 17, 2020, https://www.cbc.ca/news /canada/north/kami-kandola-personal-profile-1.5545798.

196   **At her order, restaurants, gyms, schools, and some offices remained closed until the territory ticked into June:** Anna Desmarais, "N.W.T. on track for Phase 2 of COVID-19 reopening plan, top doctor says," CBC News, June 3, 2020, https://www.cbc.ca/news/canada/north/nwt-phase -two-reopening-plan-1.5597510.

196   **At the end of August, a checkpoint in Hay River, close to the Alberta border, was still refusing entry to at least a dozen vehicles a day:** Paul Bickford, "Border enforcement: About a dozen vehicles a day refused permission to travel in the NWT," *NNSL Media*, August 5, 2020, https:// nnsl.com/hayriverhub/border-enforcement-about-a-dozen-vehicles-a -day-refused-permission-to-travel-in-the-nwt.

196   **As fall hit, the territory enacted mandatory mask measures at airports:** "N.W.T. to make masks mandatory inside airport terminal buildings," CBC News, October 8, 2020, https://www.cbc.ca/news/canada/north/ masks-mandatory-inside-airport-terminal-buildings-nwt-1.5755949.

197   **On April 15, Saskatchewan's far north reported its first COVID-19 case in La Loche, a Dene village that's home to about 2,800 people:** Phil Tank, "Saskatchewan's worst COVID-19 outbreak ends in La Loche," *Saskatoon Star Phoenix*, July 16, 2020, https://thestarphoenix.com/news /local-news/saskatchewans-worst-covid-19-outbreak-ends-in-la-loche.

197   **Health officials later confirmed the virus' arrival in the community was linked to travel from an oil sands camp in Alberta:** Kristy Kirkup

and Marsha McLeod, "'Alarming' COVID-19 outbreak hits northern Saskatchewan," *Globe and Mail*, May 7, 2020, https://www.theglobeandmail.com/canada/article-alarming-outbreak-hits-northern-saskatchewan.

197 **By the time the province restricted non-critical travel to the province's north eleven days later, the area accounted for twenty-five of the fifty-seven active cases:** David Giles, "Non-critical travel to northern Saskatchewan restricted due to coronavirus outbreak," Global News, April 24, 2020, https://globalnews.ca/news/6865789/non-critical-travel-northern-saskatchewan-coronavirus.

197 **More than two hundred people in La Loche got sick, and another sixty-two:** Phil Tank, "Saskatchewan's worst COVID-19 outbreak ends in La Loche," *Saskatoon Star Phoenix*, July 16, 2020, https://thestarphoenix.com/news/local-news/saskatchewans-worst-covid-19-outbreak-ends-in-la-loche.

199 **Finally, upon discovering why she was there, a nurse told her, "Oh, you don't know yet? She's died":** "Relatives, experts call for accountability in wake of Joyce Echaquan's death," *The Current*, October 1, 2020, https://www.cbc.ca/radio/thecurrent/the-current-for-oct-1-2020-1.5745953/relatives-experts-call-for-accountability-in-wake-of-joyce-echaquan-s-death-1.5746359#:~:text=Joyce%20Echaquan%2C%20a%2037%2Dyear,hour%20drive%20from%20her%20community.

199 **Indigenous people know all too well that, despite politicians' protestations otherwise:** Claire Loewen, "Quebec premier's apology did not win the trust of Joyce Echaquan's family, says Atikamekw grand chief," CBC News, October 7, 2020, https://www.cbc.ca/news/canada/montreal/joyce-echaquan-constant-awashish-legault-1.5753402.

199 **such incidents are far from rare:** Morgan Lowrie and Kelly Geraldine Malone, "Joyce Echaquan's death highlights systemic racism in healthcare, experts say," CTV News, October 4, 2020, https://www.ctvnews.ca/health/joyce-echaquan-s-death-highlights-systemic-racism-in-health-care-experts-say-1.5132146.

200 **Those on reserve had a virus case rate four times lower than the general population, with three times fewer fatalities and a 30 per cent higher recovery rate:** Lisa Richardson and Allison Crawford, "COVID-19 and the decolonization of Indigenous public health," *CMAJ* 192, no. 38 (September 21, 2020), https://www.cmaj.ca/content/192/38/E1098#:~:text=In%20contrast%20to%20predictions%20early,related%20to%20poorer%20health%20outcomes.

200 **And in La Loche, the outbreak finally ended:** Bonnie Allen, "Largest outbreak of COVID-19 in an Indigenous community in Canada offers important lessons," CBC News, September 29, 2020, https://www.cbc.ca

/news/canada/saskatchewan/outbreak-covid-19-indigenous-community
-lessons-1.5737126.

203 **Around that time, four COVID-19 outbreaks shook Toronto Western,
spreading to nineteen patients and forty-six staff members:** Jennifer
Yang and May Warren, "COVID-19 outbreaks at Toronto Western
Hospital cause disruption, confusion as 65 patients and staff test
positive," *Toronto Star,* May 4, 2020, https://www.thestar.com/news/gta
/2020/05/04/covid-19-outbreaks-at-toronto-western-hospital-cause
-disruption-confusion-as-65-patients-and-staff-test-positive.html.

206 **and, carried on those twin waves like flotsam, a national increase in
drug overdoses and substance abuse:** "Canada's other health crisis: As
overdoses surge, officials call on government to decriminalize illicit
drugs," *Washington Post,* August 16, 2020, https://www.washingtonpost
.com/world/the_americas/canada-drug-overdose-coronavirus/2020/08
/15/559dabbe-dcd9-11ea-b4af-72895e22941d_story.html.

206 **in suicide and self-harm:** "Warning signs: More Canadians thinking
about suicide during pandemic," Canadian Mental Health Association,
June 25, 2020, https://cmha.ca/news/warning-signs-more-canadians-
thinking-about-suicide-during-pandemic.

207 **When she took the job in January 2019:** Kashmala Fida, "Leading with
her heart: Long before COVID-19, Deena Hinshaw was making an
impression," CBC News, April 1, 2020, https://www.cbc.ca/news/canada
/edmonton/profile-deena-hinshaw-alberta-chief-medical-officer-of
-health-1.5515572.

208 **And, admittedly, she's said something similar in several other
interviews:** Geoff McMaster, "Deena Hinshaw: The making of an unlikely
folk hero," *folio,* May 7, 2020, https://www.folio.ca/deena-hinshaw-the
-making-of-an-unlikely-folk-hero; https://www.mountainviewtoday.ca
/local-news/albertas-top-doctor-sorry-for-confusion-over-back-to
-school-order-update-2678833.

Eight: A High Toll

212 **The next night, one of the facility's residents, an eighty-three-year-
old man, died, becoming Canada's first COVID-19 death:** Mike Hagar
and Andrea Woo, "How the coronavirus took North Vancouver's Lynn
Valley Care Centre," *Globe and Mail,* March 21, 2020, https://www
.theglobeandmail.com/canada/article-how-the-coronavirus-took-north
-vancouvers-lynn-valley-care-centre.

215 **Here, long-term care residents accounted for 81 per cent of all
COVID-19 deaths; the average in other countries stood at 38 per cent:**
"CIHI snapshot: Pandemic experience in the long-term care sector,"

Canadian Institute for Health Information, 2020, https://www.cihi.ca/sites/default/files/document/covid-19-rapid-response-long-term-care-snapshot-en.pdf.

215 **The disaster rumbled under the radar until, that same month, the Canadian Armed Forces (CAF) released a report on five care homes in Ontario**: "JTFC observations in long-term care facilities in Ontario," 4th Canadian Division Joint Task Force, May 2020, http://s3.documentcloud.org/documents/6928480/OP-LASER-JTFC-Observations-in-LTCF-in-On.pdf.

216 **as the CAF put it, "to provide humanitarian relief and medical support"**: Adam Carter, "Military report reveals what sector has long known: Ontario's nursing homes are in trouble," CBC News, May 27, 2020, https://www.cbc.ca/news/canada/toronto/military-long-term-care-home-report-covid-ontario-1.5585844.

218 **all so they wouldn't be treated, as one former student put it during the pandemic, like "glorified shit cleaners"**: Nicholas Keung and Jason Miller, "Until COVID-19 hit, PSWs went virtually unnoticed. That's changed and some say we have a lot of lessons to learn about the trials they face," *Toronto Star*, May 1, 2020, https://www.thestar.com/news/gta/2020/04/30/until-covid-19-hit-psws-received-almost-no-recognition-thats-changed.html.

218 **In May, she wrote an op-ed in *Maclean's* arguing that the national regulation of PSWs could have largely prevented the unfolding tragedy in long-term care facilities**: Laura Bulmer, "How the pandemic would have been different if PSWs were regulated," *Maclean's*, May 21, 2020, https://www.macleans.ca/opinion/how-the-pandemic-would-have-been-different-if-psws-were-regulated.

219 **The result of all this is a workforce that is majority women, many of whom are racialized or new to Canada**: "Re-imagining long-term residential care in the COVID-19 crisis," Canadian Centre for Policy Alternatives, April 24, 2020, https://www.policyalternatives.ca/publications/reports/re-imagining-long-term-residential-care-covid-19-crisis.

221 **By May, around nine thousand PSWs in Quebec had either refused to work or had become sick with COVID-19**: Tom Mulcair, "Quebec's coronavirus outbreak in long-term care homes could have been prevented," *Maclean's*, May 14, 2020, https://www.macleans.ca/opinion/quebecs-long-term-care-coronavirus-outbreak-could-have-been-prevented/.

221 **Fifty-one-year-old Arlene Reid died on April 27 while her daughter frantically performed CPR**: Adam Carter, "'She's a hero': Family mourns health-care worker who died after contracting COVID-19,"

CBC News, April 30, 2020, https://www.cbc.ca/news/canada/toronto
/covid-19-coronavirus-health-care-worker-death-1.5550861.

221 **Each had a shortage of PPE; her home care job provided two surgical
masks every five days:** Ibid.

222 **"I'm going to get better. Mommy is going to be okay. I'm going to walk
away from this":** Ibid.

223 **"My mom died at my house," her daughter told the** *Globe and Mail*.
"She just wanted to get better": Laura Stone, "Before a personal support
worker died from COVID-19, she was worried about a lack of PPE,
family says," *Globe and Mail*, May 1, 2020, https://www.theglobeandmail
.com/canada/article-second-ontario-personal-support-worker-dies-after
-contracting-covid-19.

227 **It had, by then, appeared in more than sixty-five thousand tweets and
references to the higher mortality rate among older people infected
with COVID-19:** Andrew Whalen, "What is 'Boomer Remover' and why
is it making people so angry?" *Newsweek*, March 13, 2020, https://www
.newsweek.com/boomer-remover-meme-trends-virus-coronavirus
-social-media-covid-19-baby-boomers-1492190.

227 **Around that same time, WHO director-general Tedros Adhanom
Ghebreyesus slammed countries that were responding slowly, or
poorly, to the virus:** "WHO emergencies coronavirus press conference,"
World Health Organization, March 9, 2020, https://www.who.int/docs
/default-source/coronaviruse/transcripts/who-audio-emergencies
-coronavirus-press-conference-full-09mar2020-(1).pdf?sfvrsn=d2684d61_2.

227 **"Covid-19 didn't matter much if it was a scourge only among the old":**
Louise Aronson, "'Covid-19 kills only old people.' Only?" *New York
Times*, March 22, 2020, https://www.nytimes.com/2020/03/22/opinion
/coronavirus-elderly.html.

228 **Days into his country's lockdown, the lieutenant governor of Texas
even suggested grandparents would be willing to sacrifice themselves
for the country's economic future:** Adrianna Rodriguez, "Texas'
lieutenant governor suggests grandparents are willing to die for US
economy," *USA Today*, March 24, 2020, https://www.usatoday.com/story
/news/nation/2020/03/24/covid-19-texas-official-suggests-elderly
-willing-die-economy/2905990001.

228 **"If grandma dies in a nursing home at age 81, that's tragic and that's
terrible, also the life expectancy in the United States is 80":** David
Wallace-Wells, "COVID-19 targets the elderly. Why don't our prevention efforts?" *New York Magazine*, May 13, 2020, https://nymag.com
/intelligencer/2020/05/covid-targets-the-elderly-why-dont-our
-prevention-efforts.html.

228 **Ukraine's ex–health minister said those over aged sixty-five were already "corpses":** Paul Nash and Phillip W. Schnarrs, "Coronavirus shows how ageism is harmful to health of older adults," The Conversation, June 15, 2020, https://theconversation.com/coronavirus -shows-how-ageism-is-harmful-to-health-of-older-adults-138249.

229 **"It is revealing that the younger adults who have died from complica- tions of COVID-19 throughout the world have often generated long and in-depth media reports," wrote the authors:** Sarah Fraser, et al., "Ageism and COVID-19: What does our society's response say about us?" *Age and Ageing* 49 (May 2020): 692–95, doi.org/10.1093/ageing/afaa097.

229 **What's more, unlike in other countries, where men account for a greater portion of COVID-19 deaths, the sheer number of long-term care deaths here has tipped the gender balance:** David Seglins, Andreas Wesley, and Roberto Rocha, "We looked at every confirmed COVID-19 case in Canada. Here's what we found," CBC News, September 23, 2020, https://www.cbc.ca/news/canada/public-health-agency-of-canada -covid-19-statistics-1.5733069.

230 **By the next month, long-term care deaths would encompass 97 per cent of all deaths in Nova Scotia:** "CIHI snapshot: Pandemic experience in the long-term care sector," Canadian Institute for Health Information, 2020, https://www.cihi.ca/sites/default/files/document/covid-19-rapid -response-long-term-care-snapshot-en.pdf.

230 **And by June, fifty-three residents at Northwood had died from the virus:** Shaina Luck, "Inside the Halifax high-rise at the centre of a Canadian COVID-19 tragedy," *CBC News*, June 4, 2020, https://ww.cbc .ca/news/canada/nova-scotia/northwood-halifax-covid-19-what -happened-1.5596220.

231 **And for twenty years, until she was diagnosed with dementia, she sang with the Nova Scotia Mass Choir:** Elizabeth Chiu, "Nova Scotia cabinet minister reflects on losing his trailblazing mom to COVID-19," CBC News, May 7, 2020, https://www.cbc.ca/news/canada/nova-scotia /northwood-halifax-covid-19-what-happened-1.5596220.

231 **By fall, cases began to reappear in long-term care centres—including in some that had previously quelled their outbreaks:** Simon Little, "New COVID-19 outbreak at Vancouver care home where 13 died," Global News, September 30, 2020, https://globalnews.ca/news/7370279 /new-haro-park-centre-coronavirus-outbreak.

231 **By October, resident cases in Ontario long-term care homes were approaching April numbers at 159 virus-positive patients; at 199, staff cases had already surpassed their April tallies:** Kenyon Wallace, "It's April all over again. A look at the numbers shows Ontario could be on

the brink of another long-term-care catastrophe," *Toronto Star,* October 16, 2020, https://www.thestar.com/news/canada/2020/10/16/its-april-all-over-again-a-look-at-the-numbers-shows-ontario-could-be-on-the-brink-of-another-long-term-care-catastrophe.html.

231 **The province asked the Red Cross to help in several homes, just as the disaster relief organization had done over the summer in Quebec:** Paola Loriggio, "Ontario deciding which long-term care homes to get Red Cross support," *Toronto Star,* October 13, 2020, https://www.thestar.com/news/gta/2020/10/13/ontario-deciding-which-long-term-care-homes-to-get-red-cross-support.html.

233 **The reported rate of false negatives ranges between 2 and 37 per cent:** Robert H. Schmerling, "Which test is best for COVID-19?" Harvard Health Publishing, August 10, 2020, https://www.health.harvard.edu/blog/which-test-is-best-for-covid-19-2020081020734.

234 **A later antibody test, which uses a person's blood and can show whether they had the virus in the past, came back positive:** May Warren, "Here's who's eligible for a COVID-19 antibody test in Ontario," *Toronto Star,* September 11, 2020, https://www.thestar.com/news/gta/2020/09/11/heres-whos-eligible-for-a-covid-19-antibody-test-in-ontario.html.

Nine: Recovery

238 **Live attenuated vaccines have been used to fend off everything from the rotavirus to measles, mumps, and rubella:** "Vaccine types," U.S. Department of Health and Human Services, https://www.vaccines.gov/basics/types.

239 **"However," as a July 2020 article in *Nature Materials* noted, "certain limitations are associated with several of these platforms that make them less amenable to fast vaccine production in a pandemic":** Debby van Riel and Emmir de Wit, "Next generation vaccine platforms for COVID-19," *Nature Materials* 19 (2020): 810–12, https://www.nature.com/articles/s41563-020-0746-0.

240 **that is, if the world keeps producing possible global pandemics, which it sadly seems likely to:** Susanne Rauch, Edith Jasny, Kim E. Schmidt, Benjamin Petsch, "New vaccine technologies to combat outbreak situations," *Frontiers in Immunology* 19 (September 2018), https://doi.org/10.3389/fimmu.2018.01963.

240 **One such next-gen platform is called a viral vector-based vaccine, which is based off the same platform as the Canadian-made Ebola vaccine:** "Safety of Ebola virus vaccines," World Health Organization (2019), https://www.who.int/vaccine_safety/committee/topics/ebola/Jul_2019/en/.

244 **"It doesn't have any disinfectant in it, does it?":** Cecie Elnicki, interviewed by John Moore, Newstalk 1010, April 30, 2020, https://omny .fm/shows/newstalk1010/cecie-elnicki-with-john-moore#description.

245 **Complicating it all further, most of the next-generation platforms have never been licensed for any pathogen:** Nicole Lurie, Melanie Saville, Richard Hatchett, and Jane Halton, "Developing Covid-19 vaccines at pandemic speed," *New England Journal of Medicine* 382 (2020): 1969–73, https://www.nejm.org/doi/full/10.1056/NEJMp2005630.

245 **In 1717, Lady Mary Wortley Montagu, the wife of the British ambassador to Turkey, witnessed her first variolation in Constantinople:** Alexandra Flemming, "The origins of vaccination," *Nature Research* (September 2020), https://www.nature.com/articles /d42859-020-00006-7.

246 **A precursor to vaccination, the process involved inserting a thread into the pustule of a person infected with a mild case of smallpox:** Frank M. Snowden, *Epidemics and Society: From the Black Death to the Present* (Yale University Press, 2019), 105.

249 **In October 2020, for example,** *Nature Medicine* **released:** Joanne Laucius, "Vaccine hesitancy and Covid-19: how many will stay on the fence?," *Ottawa Citizen*, December 18, 2020, https://ottawacitizen.com /news/local-news/vaccine-hesitancy-and-covid-19-how-many-will-stay -on-the-fence; Angus Reid Institute, December 14, 2020, http://angusreid .org/canada-covid-vaccine-december/; Jeffrey V. Lazarus et al., "A global survey of potential acceptance of a COVID-19 vaccine," *Nature Medicine*, October 20, 2020, https://www.nature.com/articles/s41591-020-1124-9.

249 **In fact, after the discovery of penicillin in 1945, it took nearly another forty years fore the first antiviral drug to be licensed:** Dorothy H. Crawford, *Viruses: A Very Short Introduction* (Oxford University Press, 2011), 121.

250 **Remdesivir is an antiviral that can cut recovery times by five days:** Marilynn Marchione, "FDA approves first COVID-19 drug: the antiviral remdesivir," CTV News, October 2020, https://www.ctvnews.ca/health /coronavirus/fda-approves-first-covid-19-drug-the-antiviral -remdesivir-1.5156780.

251 **Canada recorded its first case on April 26, 2009:** "The H1N1 Flu in Ontario: A report by Ontario's Chief Medical Officer of Health," Ministry of Health and Long-Term Care, September 2009, http://www.health.gov .on.ca/en/ccom/flu/h1n1/pro/docs/oh9100_report.pdf.

251 **and its first aseltamivir-resistant case scant weeks later on July 21:** "First Tamiflu-resistant H1N1 case found in Canada," CTV News, July 22, 2009, https://www.ctvnews.ca/first-tamiflu-resistant-h1n1-case-found-in -canada-1.419146.

252 **In other words, interferons won't kill a virus directly, but they will trigger a defence response in other cells, preventing the virus from replicating within them:** Marco De Andrea, Raffaella Ravera, Daniela Gioia, Marisa Gariglio, and Santo Landolfo, "The interferon system: An overview," *European Journal of Paediatric Neurology* 6 (2002): A41–A46, https://doi.org/10.1053/ejpn.2002.0573.

252 **who immediately set up an exploratory study using interferons to treat virus patients at a hospital in Wuhan:** Qiong Zhou et al., "Interferon-a2b treatment for COVID-19," *Frontiers in Immunology* (May 2020), https://doi.org/10.3389/fimmu.2020.01061.

253 **She has been asked, and has sometimes agreed, to join the scientific advisory boards of several pharmaceutical companies:** "BetterLife Pharma announces apointment of Dr. Eleanor Fish, a leading expert on interferon activity against Covid-19, to its advisory board," Cision, May 2020, https://www.newswire.ca/news-releases/betterlife-pharma -announces-appointment-of-dr-eleanor-fish-a-leading-expert-on -interferon-activity-against-covid-19-to-its-advisory-board-888781569.html.

255 **The study was so successful, she's now helping local health authorities develop an interferon clinic:** "U of T's immunologist's new drug shows promise in treating Ebola," *U of T News*, March 2017, https://www .utoronto.ca/news/u-t-immunologist-s-new-drug-shows-promise -treating-ebola.

257 **For example, Senior's former organization, YWCA Canada, and the Institute for Gender and the Economy at the University of Toronto's Rotman School of Management jointly released a feminist economic recovery plan in July 2020:** Anjum Saltana and Carmina Ravanera, "A feminist economic recovery plan for Canada," YWCA Canada, July 2020, https://www.feministrecovery.ca.

259 **And in June, the Vancouver Police Department said there had been a 600 per cent increase:** Robin Gill, "Asian communities across Canada report rising racist behaviour during COVID-19 crisis," Global News, June 7, 2020, https://globalnews.ca/news/7033253/coronavirus-asian -racism-crisis-canada.

Epilogue

266 **That day, Ontario, my home province, recorded the highest number of new COVID-19 cases in a single day since the beginning of the pandemic:** "Tracking Ontario's 102,378 cases of COVID-19," CTV News, March 2, 2020, https://toronto.ctvnews.ca/tracking-ontario-s-105-501 -cases-of-covid-19-1.4834821.

266 **Around that time, Canada itself passed a grim milestone of two hundred thousand total cases:** "Canada kicked off EU's safe country

list due to high number of coronavirus cases," Global News, October 21, 2020, https://globalnews.ca/news/7410196/eu-safe-country-list -canada-kicked-off-coronavirus; "EU removes Canadians from a list of approved travellers because of COVID-19," CBC News, October 21, 2020, https://www.cbc.ca/news/business/eu-travel-canada-1.5770782.

266 **By the end of the month, the virus had killed over ten thousand people in Canada**: David Lao and Hannah Jackson, "Over 10,000 people in Canada have died from coronavirus," Global News, October 27, 2020, https://globalnews.ca/news/7421380/canada-coronavirus-10k-death-toll; "Statement from the Chief Public Health Officer of Canada," Public Health Agency of Canada, October 29, 2020, https://www.canada.ca/en /public-health/news/2020/10/statement-from-the-chief-public-health -officer-of-canada-on-october-29-2020.html.

266 **People cancelled Thanksgiving plans, then Halloween trick-or-treating**: Emerald Bensadoun, "Fewer Canadians to hand out Halloween candy, trick or treat this year, poll says," Global News, October 29, 2020, https://globalnews.ca/news/7427356/ipsos-poll-halloween-canada.

267 **Winter holidays seemed up in the air, and even Trudeau suggested Christmas might be cancelled**: Ryan Tumilty, "The COVID-19 pandemic 'really sucks,' and also Christmas is now in jeopardy, Trudeau warns," *National Post*, October 27, 2020, https://nationalpost.com/news /politics/the-covid-19-pandemic-really-sucks-and-christmas-is-now-in -jeopardy-trudeau-warns.

267 **In Canada, cases among twentysomethings have surged, surpassing the number of cases of those in the eighty-plus age range near the end of August**: Dave Seglins, Andreas Wesley, and Roberto Rocha, "We looked at every confirmed COVID case in Canada. Here's what we found," CBC News, September 23, 2020, https://www.cbc.ca/news/canada/public -health-agency-of-canada-covid-19-statistics-1.5733069.

267 **In England, it found, a person aged fifty-five to sixty-four "who gets infected with SARS-CoV-2 faces a fatality risk that is more than 200 times higher than the annual risk of dying in a fatal car accident"**: Stuart Thomson, "Study confirms massive age differences in COVID-19 death rates, middle-aged hit harder than thought," *National Post*, July 30, 2020, https://nationalpost.com/health/study-confirms-massive-age -differences-in-covid-19-death-rates-middle-aged-hit-harder-than-thought.

267 **"Fortunately, your government has already shown us what needs to be done"**: Bryce Hoye, "Lock down Manitoba because 'it's too late' for targeted restrictions, doctors urge government," CBC News, October 30, 2020, https://www.cbc.ca/news/canada/manitoba/manitoba-doctors -call-for-provincewide-shutdown-covid19-1.5783335; "Doctors call for

province-wide lockdown: An open letter," *Winnipeg Free Press*, October 30. 2020, https://www.winnipegfreepress.com/opinion/analysis/doctors-call -for-provincewide-lockdown-572920561.html.

271 **At the end of October, Theresa Tam released her annual report on the state of public health in Canada:** "Chief public health officer of Canada's report on the state of public health in Canada in 2020," October 2020.

272 **It's a flip on the "we're all in it together" line and one that feels not only more honest but more helpful. At a later press conference:** Rachel Aiello, "Canada's top doctor calls for 'structural change' to address COVID-19 inequities," CTV News, October 28, 2020, https:// www.ctvnews.ca/health/coronavirus/canada-s-top-doctor-calls-for -structural-change-to-address-covid-19-inequities-1.5164415.

272 **"Why can't we have those governance structures beyond the crisis and into recovery?":** Theresa Tam as quoted by Rachel Aiello, "Canada's top doctor calls for 'structural change' to address COVID-19 inequities," CTV News, October 28, 2020, https://www.ctvnews.ca/health/ coronavirus/canada-s-top-doctor-calls-for-structural-change-to- address-covid-19-inequities-1.5164415.

Acknowledgements

Though it may often feel like it, writing a book is anything but a solitary endeavour. With *Women of the Pandemic*, I was lucky to have a brilliant, creative, and endlessly supportive team. To everyone at McClelland & Stewart who helped bring this book into being, thank you. An especially big thank you to my editor, Jenny Bradshaw, who graciously took many scattered phone calls as I worked through the ideas, structure, and scope of this book, and offered patient, considered insight in return—not to mention her deft and thoughtful editing of everything that eventually landed on the page. Thank you to publisher Jared Bland for trusting me with this vital, fascinating project. Thank you to Kristin Cochrane for seeing the necessity of a project like this.

I'm also incredibly grateful to designer Andrew Roberts for a vivid, eye-catching cover; to copy-editor Tara Tovell for her much-needed fine-tooth comb and sharp questions; to proofreader Erin Kern for her close read of every word and keen ability to vanquish typos; to editorial intern Trudy Fegan for helping to wrangle the many, many footnotes; and to publicity manager Ruta Liormonas, whose enthusiasm for the project built the platform for these women's stories to be shared. I could not ask for a smarter, more encouraging team and I feel very fortunate to have worked on *Women of the Pandemic* with all of you.

To my agent, Hilary McMahon, thank you for being both such a steadfast cheerleader and reality check, and for always finding the perfect home for my words. And to my family and friends—there's no way I would have made it through 2020 without your phone calls and texts, handmade care packages, Zoom craft sessions and card nights, socially distanced park boxing workouts, and many walks through both Toronto's tree-lined trails and most bougie neighbourhoods. Add writing a book to that unprecedented year and, well, I don't think I can thank you all enough for all the love you sent my way. I'm grateful for your check-ins, your laughter, your kindness, and your persistent reminders to leave my desk once in a while. It was a tough year in so many ways, and I'm grateful I journeyed through it with so many extraordinary people, apart but together.

But, most of all, thank you to everybody who shared their stories for this book. I appreciate your generosity, your vulnerability, and your openness. You carried us all through this sometimes-terrible, sometimes-inspiring, always-transformative time. You led and you sacrificed, and did everything you could to keep us all safe, even when it meant putting yourself in danger. To all the women of the pandemic: thank you. I wish that I could tell all of your stories; we need to hear them. Though I've tried the best I can to put your experiences into words, I believe the truth is that we owe you all more than we can express. May we begin to move forward with hope, kindness, compassion, and community—in a way that can honour what you gave us.